S T U D E N T W O R K B O O K

for

Introduction to Communication
Sciences and Disorders

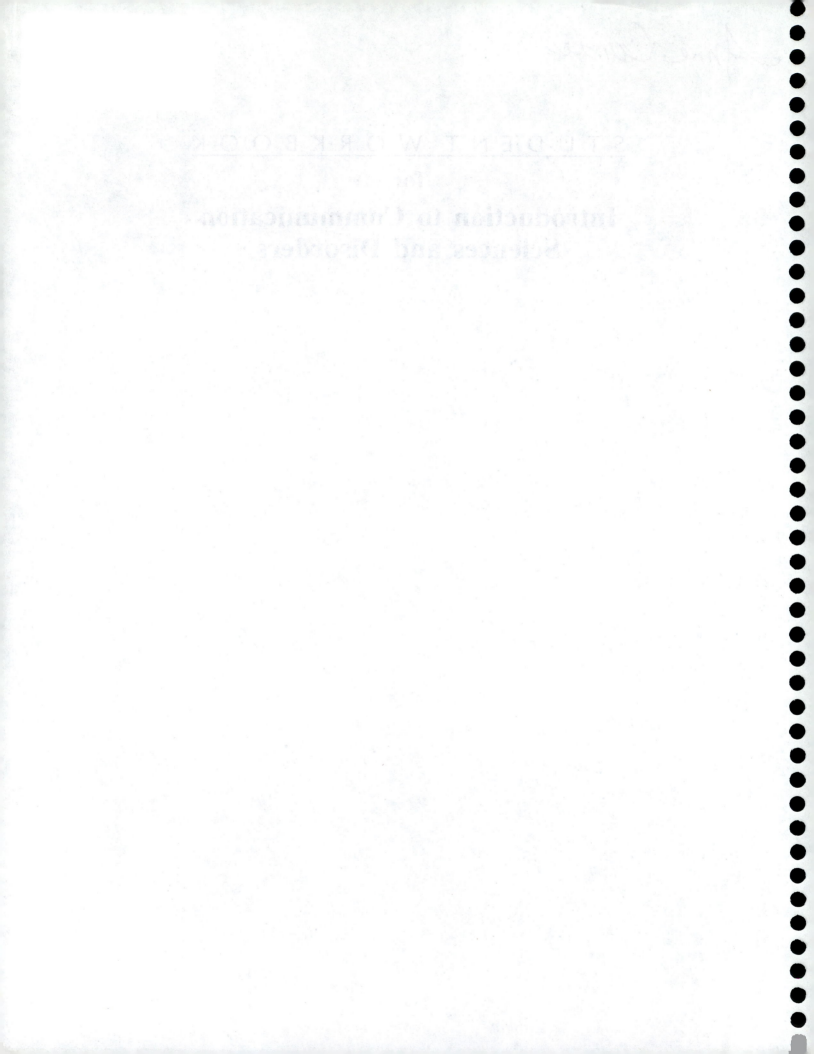

STUDENT WORKBOOK

for

Introduction to Communication Sciences and Disorders

Fred D. Minifie, Ph.D.

with
Carolyn R. Carter, M.S., and Jason L. Smith, B.A.

SINGULAR PUBLISHING GROUP, INC.
SAN DIEGO, CALIFORNIA

Singular Publishing Group, Inc.
4284 41st Street
San Diego, California 92105-1197

Typeset in 12/14 Times by ExecuStaff Composition Services
Printed in the United States of America by McNaughton & Gunn

ISBN 1-56593-361-3

CONTENTS

INTRODUCTION

The purpose of this workbook is to provide structured opportunities for students to continue to learn and expand on the information contained in the main text. Each chapter in the workbook is divided into three sections, each presenting a different level of exercise to the student.

The first section in each chapter is designed to be used as a study guide to help students further review, organize, and understand what the author presents in the text. The questions in this section are based directly on the corresponding chapter in the textbook.

The second level of exercises in the workbook is designed to help students integrate the information from the text by presenting questions that require more analytical applications of the material. These are short essay questions that may ask the student to pursue additional information to supplement the text or to provide personal interpretations of concepts to explore his or her own ideas. Although these questions can stand alone as written exercises, they may also serve as the impetus for class discussion groups or as springboards for more formal written assignments such as term papers.

The third section in each chapter provides suggestions for activities that might be performed by individual students, laboratory sections, or the class as a whole. These activities provide alternatives to traditional writing assignments and are designed to help students experience the topic of interest beyond the academic classroom environment.

Introduction to the Professions

RICHARD M. FLOWER, Ph.D.

STUDY GUIDE

1. **a.** A specialized area of study requiring mastery of theoretical and applied knowledge of human communication and its disorders defines the discipline of:

   _____

   b. Two different professions belong to this discipline. They are:

   (1) _____

   (2) _____

2. The work performed by the two groups of professionals named above includes three major activities. Name the three forms of work:

   a. _____

   b. _____

   c. _____

3. To perform their professional duties, speech pathologists and audiologists must gain knowledge bases in other disciplines that are closely related to human communication and its disorders. Name at least four disciplines from which speech pathologists and audiologists draw knowledge.

    a. _____

    b. _____

    c. _____

    d. _____

4. In discussing the history of communication sciences and disorders, the author states that interest in treating people with communication disorders emerged from two perspectives. Name two broad disciplines which provided the initial impetus for developing services for children and adults with communication disorders. Their influence is still evident in the settings in which speech-language pathologists and audiologists work today:

    a. _____

    b. _____

5. The American Speech-Language-Hearing Association (ASHA) was formed in 1926. ASHA performs many important functions both for members of the professions and for the public. List five of ASHA's contributions:

    a. _____

    b. _____

    c. _____

    d. _____

    e. _____

6. Frequently speech-language pathologists and audiologists are closely allied in the work they each perform. However, speech-language pathology and audiology are considered separate professions. The text suggests two reasons for this separation. Discuss these two reasons and any benefits or disadvantages you see in separating speech-language pathology and audiology.

_____

_____

_____

_____

7.   **a.** What event in the 1940s triggered tremendous expansion in the discipline of communication sciences and disorders?

_____

   b. What role did the event have in the growth of the profession?

_____

_____

_____

_____

8.   In describing the scope of practice of a speech-language pathologist, the author defines seven primary functions that this profession performs. Briefly describe below the seven areas within a speech-language pathologist's scope of practice:

   a. _____

   _____

   b. _____

   _____

   c. _____

   _____

   d. _____

   _____

e. _____

_____

f. _____

_____

g. _____

_____

9. The author also provides a scope of practice description for the profession of audiology. Define six functions that fall within an audiologist's scope of practice:

a. _____

_____

b. _____

_____

c. _____

_____

d. _____

_____

e. _____

_____

f. _____

_____

10. Although professional services vary depending on the setting in which a person works, most audiologists and speech-language pathologists perform the following five professional services:

a. _____

b. _____

c. _____

d. _____

e. _____

11.   What is the difference between screening and a full diagnostic evaluation?

_____

_____

_____

_____

_____

_____

12. a. Treatment/therapy programs have three possible goals. Describe them:

(1) _____

(2) _____

(3) _____

b. Do you think all three goals are appropriate for every patient, or might some goals be better than others for some patients? Why? Can you provide some general examples to justify your response?

_____

_____

_____

_____

_____

_____

_____

13. Name two types of counseling services that speech-language pathologists and audiologists routinely perform:

a. _____

_____

b. _____

_____

14. Speech pathologists and audiologists interact frequently with professionals in other disciplines. This interaction may serve two purposes, including providing education about communication disorders in general, or sharing information about a particular patient to improve the patient's overall care. These two functions are examples of which professional service?

_____

15. Three different forms of credentialing are available to audiologists and speech-language pathologists. What are the three credentials?

a. _____

b. _____

c. _____

16. In order to obtain the most universally accepted national credentials, ASHA certification, candidates must complete the following requirements:

a. _____

b. _____

c. _____

d. _____

e. _____

f. _____

g. _____

_____

17. a. Who oversees the credentialing for work in the public schools?

_____

b. What are some disadvantages of state control over credentialing for employment in public schools?

(1) _____

_____

(2) _____

_____

(3) _____

_____

c. What might be some advantages of state control?

(1) _____

_____

(2) _____

_____

(3) _____

_____

18. a. What is significant about the rights granted by state licensure?

_____

_____

_____

b. Does your state have licensure? If so, what are the requirements to obtain a license?

_____

_____

_____

_____

_____

_____

19. a. What is the largest work setting for speech-language pathologists?

_____

b. What is the second largest setting for professionals in communication disorders?

_____

20. a. The majority of speech-language pathologists who work in schools perform "designated services." What is meant by this term?

_____

_____

_____

b. What are two more examples of school settings in which speech-language pathologists work?

(1) _____

(2) _____

21. a. What is the role of the speech-language pathologist in an acute-inpatient hospital setting?

_____

_____

b. How does this work differ from that in a longer term setting such as a rehabilitation service?

_____

_____

_____

_____

22.   The following word puzzle contains the names of 16 examples of health and community facilities in which speech-language pathologists and audiologists work. See how many you can find.

```
H O M E H E A L T H A G E N C I E S X P A C
G M E N T A L H E A L T H C E N T E R S O S
N O D P R L U E Z H T H K A I D U B L A A E
I Q I N F A N T T O D D L E R U G H A J L N
V U C U S O A L N P C R R O W S Y F I H R I
I A A B A P Z I A K U O R N N T H K G Y E O
L P L Y E S O T O B E B U N I R K S C E N R
T R G H D E I H R E H H L K F I P L Y M O C
N I R S A I R S S M E N T I S A P Y H N O E
E V O C D T L O U K T D A E C L U I I H P N
D A U S Z I X P O U R T L G A H O U T R O T
N T P H U S L B C I A O J F K E E S P E C E
E E P I O R J A U D T H W E R A O A L K F R
P P R R O E L N G U S T O B R L K J L F J S
E R A Z W V A P R W D I U T A T O R D T A U
D A C L O I T F J N A D H A R H T H E R H P
N C T C O N I L O U E A Y S W A E R O P F J
I T I O J U V E K L H F F O P L R R A S W E
R I C H I L D C A R E C E N T E R S O L J F
T C E M A T T E M N O E E K S J P U L K C Z
F E S R E D N E F F O E L I N E V U J C D E
```

Answers:

_____   _____

_____   _____

_____   _____

_____   _____

_____   _____

_____   _____

_____   _____

_____   _____

23. University clinics serve two major roles. What are they?

a. _____

b. _____

24. Speech-language pathologists and audiologists often work closely with other professionals. In the exercise that follows, match the name of each professional with the services provided by his or her discipline.

___ Pediatrician	**A.**	Provide diagnosis and treatment for any medical condition
___ Orthodontist	**B.**	Ear-Nose-Throat physician
	C.	Physician specializing in care of children
___ Occupational Medicine	**D.**	Diagnose/treat central nervous system deficits
___ Otolaryngologist	**E.**	Work to repair anatomic deficits such as cleft palate
___ Psychologist	**F.**	Work with job related injuries
___ Neurologist	**G.**	Primary health care providers in many urban and rural areas
___ Social Worker	**H.**	Treat dental malocclusions that affect speech production
___ Vocational Counselor	**I.**	Work with a patient's posture, ambulation, and limb mobility
___ Physical Therapist	**J.**	Help patients to master daily living activities (e.g., eating and bathing)
___ Physician	**K.**	Providing assistance in job placement
	L.	Provide evaluation of cognitive abilities and diagnose and treat emotional problems
___ Occupational Therapist	**M.**	Assist patients in finding needed resources and services, including economic support
___ Public Health Nurse		
___ Plastic Surgeon		

25. It is becoming more and more common in schools to place children with disabilities in classes offering the greatest amount of contact with normally developing children. The term for the environment created by this practice is:

_____

ESSAY QUESTIONS

1. In this chapter, particularly in the examples accompanying the definitions of the professions, the author presents many examples of the settings and nature of work in which speech-language pathologists and audiologists can be found. Select two of these examples which interest you. Imagine yourself as that professional. Describe in detail the settings, the patients you might see, and the other professionals with whom you would work. Why does each setting interest you?

2. Several times the author mentions the role of professionals in performing research in communication sciences and disorders. Why do you think research is so important in the discipline?

3. The author begins the chapter by stating how devastating an impact communication disorders can have on people's lives. Why do you think this is so? Describe an example of this impact based on your own experience or from illustrations in the text.

4. The author mentions helping people with accent reduction as falling within the scope of practice of a speech-language pathologist. However, this has been a controversial issue because accents and dialects are variations in speech and language, not necessarily disorders of speech and language. Take a moment to think about working with people who speak languages foreign to you, or people with different accents or dialects. Do you think they should be "treated"? Under what conditions? What special skills might the clinician need? Offer your opinion on this controversy!

5. Another area of controversy concerns models of treatment for children in schools. Should children be pulled out of their classrooms several times a week for treatment in the speech-language pathologist's office? Or should the clinician treat children within the context of the classroom? List some advantages and disadvantages for the pull-out model and the model supporting treatment in the classroom. Consider this issue from perspectives of the clinician and the child, as well as from the perspectives of the teacher and the rest of the class.

ACTIVITIES

1. Observe a speech-language pathologist or audiologist in any setting that interests you. Based on your observations, describe the following:

   a. The setting
   b. The patient and his or her disorder
   c. The types of activities the clinician did with the patient
   d. The goals of the patient
   e. Any suggestions you might have if you had been seeing the patient
   f. Did this setting interest you? Why or why not?

2. Pretend that you are a speech-language pathologist working in a hospital on the acute care ward. Your patient is a 30-year-old male who has suffered a brain injury. The man does not appear able to talk or write, yet he seems to be aware of what is going on around him. You would like to try to find a way for him to communicate. Keeping in mind that he cannot talk or write, what other alternative models of communication can you suggest that might provide a way for this patient to share his needs and thoughts with the people around him in the hospital? Be creative and share your ideas with others in the class. There is no right or wrong answer so suggest anything that might work!

3. Pretend that you are an audiologist. Your patient is a 55-year-old female who has suffered a moderate hearing loss. Although she has a hearing aid, she is not completely satisfied with it and wants some suggestions on how to further improve her communication and understanding of other people. She is very active in family gatherings and social clubs, so successful communication is important to her. What ideas do you have about how to help her? What might she try? What are some suggestions for her family and friends? What strategies could be implemented to help her remain active even with her hearing loss? Again, there are no right or wrong answers. Any idea is a good one, so give it a try. Consider technology, situational modifications, education—anything goes!

Communication and Communication Disorders in a Multicultural Society

ORLANDO L. TAYLOR, PH.D.

STUDY GUIDE

Cultural Diversity in the United States

1. What claims can be made regarding communication and communication disorders when cultural considerations are taken into account?

    a. _____

    _____

    b. _____

    _____

    c. _____

_____

_____

2. Considering the data presented in the chapter, what seems to be the general trend in the United States with regard to cultural population proportions?

_____

_____

_____

_____

3. These differential rates of growth imply that cultural diversity will _____ in the United States in the years ahead.

4. By what year do demographers project that White Americans will represent less than 50% of the population in the United States?

_____

After that year, it is projected that the largest majority of the population will be people of color.

5. The American Speech-Language-Hearing Association has established several policies dedicated to improving the cultural sensitivity of its membership. Name two such policies:

a. _____

_____

_____

b. _____

_____

_____

The Nature of Culture

6. What does the concept of **culture** encompass?

   _____

   _____

   _____

   _____

7. What are the fundamental differences between the terms **race** and **culture**?

   _____

   _____

   _____

   _____

8. Stereotypes and overgeneralizations can often be attributed to a lack of under-

   standing of _____ .

9. Many cultures may exist within a single _____

   _____

10. Answer **true** or **false** to each of the following statements about experiences with other cultures.

    a. _____ Feelings of apprehension, loneliness, and lack of confidence are uncommon when visiting or experiencing another culture.

    b. _____ Differences between cultures are often perceived as threatening.

    c. _____ What is logical and important in a particular culture may seem irrational and unimportant to an outsider.

    d. _____ One's own sense of cultural identity often is not evident until one encounters another culture.

    e. _____ Understanding another culture is a continuous process.

Communication and Culture

11. Briefly describe **communication competence.**

_____

_____

_____

_____

12. Can someone be tested for "absolute" communication competence? How (or why not)?

_____

_____

_____

_____

13. Name at least six communicative acts that appear to be influenced by culture.

_____

a. _____

b. _____

c. _____

d. _____

e. _____

f. _____

g. _____

h. _____

14. In this chapter, Taylor argued that culturally valid assessment procedures for use by speech-language pathologists should recognize that:

a. _____

_____

_____

_____

b. _____

_____

_____

_____

15. Taylor also suggested that, during clinical treatment, clinicians should:

a. _____

_____

_____

_____

b. _____

_____

_____

_____

c. _____

_____

_____

_____

d. _____

_____

_____

_____

e. _____

_____

_____

_____

ESSAY QUESTIONS

1. Briefly describe the interdependency of language and culture.

_____

_____

_____

_____

_____

_____

2. What is the difference between a speech community and a group of people who all speak the same language?

_____

_____

_____

_____

_____

_____

_____

_____

3. What is the **Creole** theory of the genesis of dialects?

_____

_____

_____

_____

_____

_____

4. When comparing different cultural communities, what can be said about similarities and differences in the process of language acquisition?

_____

_____

_____

_____

_____

_____

ACTIVITIES

1. To help bring into focus the incredible growth of cultural diversity in the United States, determine the ethnic makeup of a particular region or institution you are familiar with. Good sources may include newspapers, government publications, or other institutional publications. How does the present situation differ from that of your parents' generation? What do your answers mean with respect to the evolution of the "average" SLP/Audiology client (clinician)?

2. When attempting to learn more about another culture, it often helps to "put yourself in their shoes"—basically, attempt to see the world through their eyes. Not only do we get a better idea of what they believe defines their culture, but we also get an idea of how they feel about our culture, a perspective we rarely take. Using Table 2–1 in Chapter 2, choose 10–12 categories to investigate. Complete two "cultural evaluations." First, fill one out for the cultural group with which you have your primary identity, and then fill out the second sheet for a different culture. Trade the second evaluation with a partner who belongs to that culture, so that both of you have an "insider" and "outsider" evaluation of your culture. How do the two differ? Are you surprised by the results? How could these differences in the conception of your own culture cause difficulties in clinical or educational settings?

3. There are a multitude of ways to learn about another culture—whether voluntary or involuntary, accidental or intentional. List as many ways as you can by which you have learned about other cultures throughout your life. (e.g., if you have traveled in a foreign country, describe what you learned about the culture[s] you encountered.) How would you rate the "quality" of those sources? Why?

4. Survey your university's speech and hearing clinic to determine if there are assessment tools (tests, etc.) and intervention materials that have been designed specifically for Hispanic Americans, Native Americans, African Americans, or Asian Americans. Report your findings. What observations can you make about the adequacy of the materials available in your speech and hearing clinic with respect to serving a culturally diverse community of persons with communication disorders?

5. Write a paper on the importance of using culturally sensitive, or culturally adapted, materials in the delivery of clinical services to communicatively impaired patients. For example, if you are an audiology student, explain why speech discrimination testing should be done using speech stimuli appropriate to the culture and language of the patient. Similarly, if you are a student majoring in speech-language pathology, discuss the importance of culturally appropriate materials in clinical service delivery.

CHAPTER 3

Speech Perception

PATRICIA K. KUHL, Ph.D.

STUDY GUIDE

1. During child language acquisition, both nature and nurture influence the development of speech perception. Describe what is meant by the nature-nurture distinction? What are the effects of nature and the effects of nurture on language development?

_____

_____

_____

_____

_____

_____

_____

_____

_____

_____

2. Do children raised in different parts of the world appear to develop language skills in a reasonably similar pattern?

    _____

3. What are critical periods for language learning?

    _____

    _____

    _____

    _____

    _____

4. What is the "Decade of the Brain" and its relation to interests in speech and language development and speech and language perception?

    _____

    _____

    _____

    _____

    _____

5. Is speech perception solely dependent on how the brain decodes the incoming information from the speech signal?

    _____

    _____

    _____

_____

_____

_____

_____

_____

_____

6. Various acoustic features of the incoming speech signal allow the listener to make judgments about the speech sounds produced by the talker. Listed below are some definitions of acoustic features. Identify each feature in the space provided:

_____ : The location within the mouth or vocal airway where the major constriction of the airway occurred.

_____ : Whether the sound produced was a vowel, stop, fricative, nasal, etc.

_____ : Speech sounds produced with vocal fold vibration.

_____ : Speech sounds produced without vocal fold vibration.

_____ : Speech sounds produced with excessive acoustic resonance in the nasal passages.

_____ : Variations in pitch, tempo, and rhythm during speech production and perception.

_____ : Variations in the fundamental frequency or pitch of the voice over time.

7.   Why are intonation variations during speech important?

_____

_____

_____

_____

_____

_____

8.   Speech segmentation refers to:

_____

_____

9.   List four factors that make speech segmentation difficult.

a. _____

b. _____

c. _____

d. _____

10.   Define the concept of "Motherese."

_____

11.   List three prosodic features of Motherese.

a. _____

b. _____

c. _____

12. During the head-turn conditioning procedure for evaluating infant speech perception, what is the difference between a control trial and a change trial?

_____

_____

_____

_____

13. If a child looks in the direction of the electromechanical toy (reinforcer) during a control trial, it is scored as:

_____

_____

14. Which of the following answers is not true of the speech perception abilities of 6-month-old infants?

    a. They can discriminate between voiced and voiceless stops.

    b. They can discriminate among stress differences on syllables.

    c. They can discriminate among consonant and vowel categories.

    d. They perceptually organize speech sounds into phonetic categories (i.e., engage in categorical perception).

    e. They assign rudimentary meanings to real words.

    _____ is not true.

15. What is the difference between "identification" and "discrimination" of speech sounds?

_____

_____

_____

_____

_____

_____

16. One of the results of early listening experience by young children is that they appear to develop phonetic prototypes for the sounds in language(s) being used in their environment. Phonetic prototypes can be defined as:

_____

_____

_____

_____

17. Phonetic prototypes appear to have the property of being able to perceptually assimilate nearby sounds. What did the author call this phenomenon?

_____

18. Cross-language studies of the perceptual magnet effect suggest that by 6 months of age:

_____

_____

_____

_____

_____

_____

19.   What evidence exists to suggest that infants use more than just auditory input in the development of perceptual categories for speech processing?

_____

_____

_____

_____

_____

_____

ESSAY QUESTIONS

1. Discuss the difference between top-down and bottom-up processing during speech perception. Is there evidence to support both types of processing during speech perception? Give examples to support your arguments.

2. The head-turn conditioning procedure has been used in many studies investigating infant speech perception. Describe the procedures used in this research paradigm. What are the advantages or disadvantages of the head-turn conditioning procedure as compared to other approaches to the study of infant speech perception?

3. Define "perceptual constancy" and discuss the importance of this concept in the development of speech and language processing by young children.

4. What evidence exists from cross-language studies to suggest that linguistic experience is crucial to a child's development of language-specific categorization of speech sounds?

5. Discuss the theory of infant speech perception presented by the author in the final section of this chapter. Does evidence exist to support the notion that experience prior to the time that infants utter their first words influences their speech and language processing abilities? Discuss the implications of the evidence in regard to the nature-nurture argument.

ACTIVITIES

1. Observe an infant younger than 6 months of age for 15 minutes. Take notes on what the infant responds to in the environment. Keep a log of any babbled utterances the child makes.

2. Try to find a second infant from a different language culture who is the same age as the child observed in activity 1. Repeat the activity with the second child. Did you notice any differences? What were they?

3. Make a tape recording of the speech of a classmate, friend, or acquaintance. Make a transcription of the tape. Note whether there appear to be complete sentences and whether the words that are used are pronounced with "textbook" clarity. Did some of the words get garbled? Could you still understand the message? Why?

4. If your instructor can provide you with an opportunity to make a visual display of the speech waveform of the recording made in activity 3, see if you can identify the location of boundaries between individual speech sounds. Could you find them? Why or why not? If you can also display the tape on a "sound spectrograph," try to see if you can do a better job of identifying sound boundaries. Could you do it better? Why or why not? Did you find any silences between speech sounds? Between words? Between phrases? Between sentences?

5. Produce the vowel sound /æ/ as in the word *tap*. Now produce it in each of the following words: *pat, lamb, mam, pal, anger, dab,* and *rally*. Did the vowel sound the same way in all of those phonetic contexts? Why or why not?

6. This time produce the /r/ sound as in *rabbit*. Now produce the same sound in the following words, paying careful attention to the position of your tongue during the production of the /r/: *street, trip, grown, grapple, aurora borealis, rain, barn, fire,* and *cream*. Is the /r/ sound produced the same way each time, or are there several different variations of the /r/ sound? What are the implications of your experience in this activity for a theory of speech perception?

7. Listen to the speech of someone speaking a foreign language. Try to segment the speech into units. What did you observe? Did the speech pattern sound too fast? Could you segment the speech into sound units, syllables, words, phrases, sentences, or paragraphs? Make notes of what you learned from this experience.

Phonological Development and Disorders in Children

JUDITH R. STONE, Ph.D.
CAROL STOEL-GAMMON, Ph.D.

STUDY GUIDE

1. Many of the key words from this chapter are highlighted in bold text and defined in the glossary. Be sure to review these terms because they are important for understanding phonological development and disorders. These terms will be incorporated into questions throughout this study guide. Some of the words listed below are also important topics in this chapter, but they are not defined in the glossary. They are presented in italics in the text. Define each term:

    a. Phonology: _____

    _____

    b. Intonation: _____

    _____

    c. Gloss: _____

d. Transcription: _____

_____

e. Jargon: _____

_____

f. Receptive Language: _____

_____

g. Expressive Language: _____

_____

h. Homonyms: _____

_____

i. Distortions: _____

_____

j. Reduplication: _____

_____

k. Marking: _____

_____

l. Functional: _____

_____

2. In the introduction the authors describe three prerequisite abilities that children must have before they can successfully learn phonology. What are these three abilities?

a. _____

b. _____

c. _____

3. The phonological system of the language has three main components. One is provided for you below. Name the other two:

a. _____

b. The rule system that governs how speech sounds are used. _____

c. _____

4. a. As stated in the previous question, phonological rules, or the rules governing the use of speech sounds in the language, are an important part of phonology. Describe some uses of phonological rules:

(1) _____

(2) _____

(3) _____

b. Study the following examples and determine if each is or could be a word in the English language. Pay special attention to the combination of the sounds /ft/. *Hint:* Be sure to consider how the words are pronounced, not just how they are spelled. Based on these examples, can you write a phonological rule describing the use of the sound combination /ft/ in our language?

FTACK   AFTER   RAFT

Rule: _____

_____

5. One aspect of phonology is prosody which includes the stress patterns of words and sentences. Below is a list of words, each of which has more than one meaning depending on where stress is placed in the word. For each word, identify the part of speech and definition that is created when the stress is placed on the indicated syllable. (* = location of syllable boundary)

a. pro'*ject: _____

   pro*ject': _____

b. re'*fuse: _____

   re*fuse': _____

c. per'*mit: _____

per*mit': _____

d. in'*cline: _____

_____

in*cline': _____

e. Think of another example on your own that fits this pattern: _____

_____

6. Different stress patterns can also change the emphasis of entire sentences when the stress is placed on different words within the sentence. Take the following sentence:

"Susan wanted to eat dessert after going to the movie."

Which word(s) would you stress the most to create the following interpretations or prevent the following misinterpretations of this sentence?

a. Bob did not want to eat dessert after the movie: _____

b. Susan didn't want dessert after dinner: _____

c. Susan didn't want dinner after the movie: _____

d. Susan didn't have to eat dessert after the movie: _____

7. Prosody also includes the intonation (see definition in exercise 1b) of a sentence and how it helps to convey meaning in the sentence. Say the following sentence to convey the following intentions, and describe how the intonation and stress patterns change for each utterance:

I HAVE TO GO TO THE STORE TODAY.

a. Asking a question: _____

b. Simple statement of fact: _____

c. Urgent exclamation: _____

_____

8. a. When studying phonological development and disorders, researchers might look at the product of development and/or the process of development. What is the focus of attention in each of these two types of studies and what does each contribute to an understanding of phonology in children?

(1) Product of development: _____

_____

(2) Process of development: _____

_____

b. Which type of research do you think might be easier in terms of collecting and analyzing data? Why?

_____

_____

_____

c. In your opinion, is one type of research more important than the other or do they both contribute essential information for helping children with phonological disorders? Why do you think this?

_____

_____

_____

_____

9. The authors list several decisions that must be made about how to sample a child's speech when collecting data for research. The same variables must be considered when studying a child's speech in a clinical setting. Describe the three decisions suggested in the text and see if you can think of one more variable on your own that you might want to control when studying a child's speech:

a. _____

b. _____

c. _____

d. _____

10.   The phonemes of the language are often placed into categories based on their distinctive features. Three types of distinctive features are used to describe phonemes. These are listed below. Define each feature:

a. Place: _____

_____

b. Manner: _____

_____

c. Voicing: _____

11.   Even though infants do not use speech sounds in meaningful ways, they are learning things in these first few months that are important in phonological development. Describe five of the behaviors of infants that are evidence of their building a foundation for the use of speech sounds (*warning*—the fifth one is "hidden" in the chapter!):

a. _____

_____

b. _____

_____

c. _____

_____

d. _____

_____

e. _____

_____

12.   Although infants use vowels and many consonant sounds in their babbling, the three primary classes of consonants used in babbling (and in the foundation of

early words) are stops, nasals, and glides. List the specific sounds that you would expect to hear in babbling for each of these classes:

Stops   **Nasals**   **Glides**

_____   _____   _____

13.   At what age do you expect infants to begin to babble?

_____

14.   Although receptive and expressive abilities develop together, one tends to precede the other. Which develops first, expressive or receptive language?

_____

15. a. The first words spoken by children often do not sound like the adult form of the words. There are two criteria that children's utterances must meet to be considered words. What are they?

(1) _____

_____

(2) _____

_____

b. Although these early words are often very different from the adult forms and difficult for unfamiliar people to understand, what allows these words to be used by a child to communicate successfully?

_____

_____

16. a. Cluster reduction, gliding, and stopping are three examples of systematic speech sound category errors that children often make during development. What is the name for these systematic error patterns?

_____

b. List four more phonological processes children commonly use, and provide one example of each that is different from the examples in the text:

(1) _____

(2) _____

(3) _____

(4) _____

17. a. In looking for patterns in phonological development, the authors suggest that there are fairly consistent trends in development across phoneme classes, but more variability within each class. Explain what this means using examples from the text.

_____

_____

_____

_____

_____

_____

b. Why do you think some classes of sound develop later than others?

_____

_____

_____

_____

_____

_____

_____

18. a. At what age have children typically established their phonological system including mastery of most speech sounds, prosodic features, and phonological rules?

_____

b. However, children continue phonological development beyond this age in new ways as they enter school. Why is a good foundation in phonological development so important for learning new academic language skills?

_____

_____

19. When studying children to determine if they have phonological disorders, many possible explanations for their speech behavior must be ruled out before a diagnosis of a phonological disorder can be made. What are some explanations that the text provides as to why children might make speech errors or fail on tasks during an evaluation?

a. _____

_____

b. _____

_____

c. _____

_____

d. _____

_____

e. _____

_____

20. Children may exhibit phonological delays or disorders in two general forms that make them different from children who develop phonology normally. What are these two general categories of phonological disorders?

a. _____

_____

b. _____

_____

21. On the lines below, fill in the approximate ages or stages at which children reach the following hallmarks in phonological development:

a. _____ : first words are consistently intelligible to familiar adults in context

b. _____ : intelligible to strangers 75% of time

c. _____ : fully intelligible to strangers

22. Although it is not always possible to identify the etiologies of phonological disorders, some risk factors indicate an increased potential for delay or disorder. What are some possible causes of phonological disorders?

a. _____

b. _____

c. _____

d. _____

e. _____

f. _____

23. The authors state that there may be a genetic basis for some phonological disorders. Identify two pieces of evidence from the chapter that support this statement.

a. _____

b. _____

24. Speech-language pathologists have three primary responsibilities in working with children who have phonological disorders. These are diagnosis, treatment, and counseling. In the spaces provided, describe each of these three responsibilities and how the clinician completes them successfully.

a. Diagnosis: _____

_____

b. Treatment: _____

_____

c. Counseling: _____

_____

25. a. Compare and contrast the traditional approach to treatment versus the phonological systems approach:

_____

_____

_____

_____

_____

b. Which approach might be more appropriate for a 4-year-old child who consistently replaces his fricative phonemes with stops? Why?

_____

_____

_____

_____

_____

c. Which approach might be more appropriate for a 7-year-old child who distorts his /s/ sound but produces all other phonemes fairly well? Why?

_____

_____

_____

_____

_____

26. If therapy is successful, a child with a phonological disorder will:

    a. Begin to use his new patterns of speech on phonemes that are not specifically trained in therapy

    b. He will also begin to use his new speech skills at home, school, and in other settings outside of the speech therapy session.

Both of these are examples of _____

ESSAY QUESTIONS

1. Pretend that you are a clinician who will be working with a bilingual child whom you suspect may have a phonological disorder. The parents speak Spanish much more fluently than they do English. The child, your patient, seems to be equally fluent in both. Explain how this bilingualism might influence how you diagnose, treat, and counsel this child and her family. What are some variables that you might need to consider with respect to their language and culture, and what special adjustments might you need to make in your methods?

2. Describe and compare longitudinal and cross-sectional research studies. What important information does each contribute to knowledge about communication disorders? What are some disadvantages of each? Now make the same comparison for retrospective versus prospective research.

3. The authors suggest that the evaluation of a child in a clinical setting is much like the investigative process used in research. Describe how clinical diagnosis and research studies are similar in their goals, methods, and use of results. How do clinical and research activities differ in their goals, methods, and use of information?

4. Phonological development is just one component in a child's overall growth and development. Undoubtedly, a child's progress in phonological development can both influence and be influenced by growth in other domains. Describe how phonological development might interact with child development in the following areas: socialization, cognitive development, education, motor development, and language development. Discuss the interactions with each of these five domains from two perspectives:

    a. How problems in each of these domains might affect phonological development.
    b. How problems in phonological development might affect each of these five domains.

5. Hearing loss is one of the risk factors that might lead to a phonological disorder. Explain why this is and describe some of the variables that determine the impact a hearing impairment might have on phonological development.

In addition, describe how the impact of a hearing loss on phonological development and a person's use of speech sounds might vary depending on the age of onset of the hearing loss. Differentiate the impact of hearing loss at each of the following ages:

a. Congenital (at birth)

b. 2 years old

c. 5 years old

d. 15 years old

ACTIVITIES

1. The following chart organizes all of the consonant sounds of the English language according to the three distinctive features of place of articulation, manner of production, and voicing. Refer to the list of consonant sounds presented in the International Phonetic Alphabet in Table 4–1 in the text. Place each of those consonant sounds in the appropriate square in the chart according to its place and manner of articulation. Then, circle any phoneme in the chart that is voiced. Some examples are provided for you.

Manner of Production

	Stops	Fricatives	Affricates	Liquids	Nasals
Bilabial two lips					
Labiodental lips to teeth					
Interdental tongue between teeth					
Alveolar tongue behind front teeth		/s/			
Palatal tongue near hard palate				/j/	
Velar back of tongue on soft palate					
Glottal air blowing through vocal folds					

2. International Phonetic Alphabet

The International Phonetic Alphabet is a system of symbols that represents speech sounds regardless of the languages in which they occur. The phonetic alphabet containing the English speech sounds is presented in Table 4–1 in the text. Practice using this alphabet by seeing if you can translate the following words into English orthography.

a. /ʃu/: _____

b. /kætʃ/: _____

c. /ɔfɪs/: _____

d. /prɛzɪdɪnt/: _____

e. /jʌmi/: _____

f. /twɛnti/: _____

g. /aktobɚ/: _____

h. /æpəl/: _____

i. /maus/: _____

j. /kʌmpjutɚ/: _____

Now it is your turn. Write the following words in the phonetic alphabet.

a. boy: _____

b. yellow: _____

c. refrigerator: _____

d. banana: _____

e. shirt: _____

f. judge: _____

g. swing: _____

h. your name: _____

i. your city: _____

j. your age: _____

3. Observation

Observe a child who is between 2 and 5 years old. Transcribe 10 of the child's utterances in the format illustrated below. (Also see the box on page 156 in the text).

Utterance	Context	Gloss	Transcription
1	_____	_____	_____
2	_____	_____	_____
3	_____	_____	_____
4	_____	_____	_____
5	_____	_____	_____
6	_____	_____	_____
7	_____	_____	_____
8	_____	_____	_____
9	_____	_____	_____
10	_____	_____	_____

Language Development

LOIS BLOOM, Ph.D.

STUDY GUIDE

1. a. When do children begin to attend to the world around them?

_____

b. How can you tell by their behavior?

(1) _____

_____

(2) _____

_____

(3) _____

_____

(4) _____

2. Infants can communicate successfully with their environment long before they learn to use language. What are some early forms of communication that would fit into the two categories below?

Emotional expressions: _____

Motoric expressions: _____

3. a. During the first year of life, infants begin to develop the symbolic capacity that will allow them to learn and use language. What is a symbol?

_____

_____

_____

_____

b. Define the term "symbolic capacity" used in the text:

_____

_____

_____

_____

c. Now, keeping that definition of a symbolic capacity in mind, compare the following two ways in which children learn to use that symbolic capacity to communicate:

Mental symbols: _____

_____

_____

Language symbols: _____

_____

_____

_____

4. a. Bloom defines language as consisting of three main components. List and define each component:

(1) _____

_____

(2) _____

_____

(3) _____

_____

b. All of the words listed below are the ingredients which make up the three main components of language you just defined. Describe each word below and assign it to the component to which it belongs:

Syntax: _____

Semantics: _____

Pragmatics: _____

Lexicon: _____

Grammar: _____

Phonology: _____

5. If you are interested in working with children with language disorders, why is it so important to understand normal language development in children?

_____

_____

_____

_____

_____

_____

6. There are many different perspectives from which to study language development. None of these theories is better than the others. Each simply contributes a different piece of the puzzle to lead to a better understanding of the intricacies of language development. Definitions of these perspectives are presented below. Label each perspective.

_____ : Focuses on language as a social phenomenon which children learn in the context of their culture's customs and traditions.

_____ : Focuses on the perspective of the child, the abilities the child brings to the process of learning language, and the change in these abilities within the context of the overall growth of the child.

_____ : Focuses on the fully developed language of the adult and what children must learn to achieve that goal.

_____ : Focuses on the personal and interpersonal variables that are present in the child and the environment, and therefore influence language development.

7. **a.** Bloom identifies three basic theories about the world that babies are developing at the beginning of the second year of life. These theories form the basis for the semantic structure of language. List the three theories and provide an example of each:

(1) _____

_____

_____

(2) _____

_____

_____

(3) _____

_____

_____

b. An example of how these three theories affect language development is evident in children as they begin to use verbs to create simple sentences. There are three categories of verbs that correspond to the three theories above. List the three types of verbs below in the order of their typical development in children. Then provide five examples of each type of verb that children may use:

(1) _____

(2) _____

(3) _____

8. There is a rather large degree of variability in the rate at which different children develop language and reach hallmarks such as saying their first words and

sentences. There may be many reasons why children seem to follow different schedules. List some reasons for this variability in development:

a. _____

_____

b. _____

_____

c. _____

_____

d. _____

_____

9. The single-word period in language development is usually marked by two boundaries.

a. The beginning of the single-word period is signalled by:

_____ at the approximate age of _____.

b. The end of the single-word period is marked by:

_____

10. a. Many of the first words that children learn are not identified by their grammatical function because children are not using the words in sentences. Instead, these first words can be placed into three categories according to what children seem to be expressing. Name the three categories and provide five examples of each:

_____   _____   _____

_____   _____   _____

_____   _____   _____

_____   _____   _____

_____   _____   _____

b. What do you think is one of the greatest influences in determining which words a child will learn?

_____

11. In her discussion of a child's first words, Bloom states that, although language can be used as a tool to influence other people, there is a more fundamental component to learning language than these instrumental purposes. The impetus for language development is demonstrated as children talk about themselves, about what they expect to happen, and about the action they see around them. These three language behaviors are examples of what phenomenon that Bloom considers the core of language development:

_____

12. Some of the first multiple-word utterances children put together include sayings such as "go bye bye" and "all gone." Why are these not considered true acts of combining words to create sentences?

_____

_____

13. a. The early simple sentences produced by children may not be grammatically correct according to adult standards. However, there are important meaning relations among the words in each sentence. Some examples of sentences a child might say are presented below. Label the meaning relation expressed by each:

(1) pretty baby: _____

(2) Daddy shoe: _____

(3) more cookie: _____

(4) nice kitty: _____

(5) no juice: _____

b. A popular classroom illustration is the demonstration that some of these simple sentences could have more than one meaning. The child's use of grammar is not yet developed enough to ensure that his or her specific mental meaning is conveyed, and the adult often must interpret the meaning of the utterance according to the context in which it occurs. For example, a child who says "Daddy shoe" could be saying several different things. How many interpretations of this simple sentence can you provide?

(1) _____

(2) _____

(3) _____

(4) _____

c. A similar example is the multiple negative meanings conveyed by the word "no" in combination with other words in simple sentences. What are the different categories of meanings that "no" might convey?

(1) _____

(2) _____

(3) _____

14. a. Language growth in children is often monitored by measuring the average length of the sentences they say. What are the units used to measure the average length of a sentence?

_____

b. Why is this a better method for measuring language development than simply referring to the child's age?

_____

_____

_____

_____

_____

15. a. Bloom provides several illustrations of one of the "basic operating principles" of language development—synergy. New or unfamiliar language content is often learned through old language forms, and new language forms are acquired by practicing with old content. Thus, a child does not have to try to manage new forms and new content at the same time, but can integrate these piece by piece into the existing language repertoire. There are three examples of this exchange between the development of form and content in the chapter. Describe them below:

(1) _____

_____

(2) _____

_____

(3) _____

_____

b. In a related manner, children also seem to budget their resources for language. If they are challenged by newly developing language structures, they will often compensate by simplifying already acquired abilities. Describe the examples of this phenomenon provided in the chapter.

(1) _____

_____

(2) _____

(3) _____

_____

(4) _____

_____

(5) _____

_____

16. a. As children learn to use verbs in sentences, they learn to add different endings to change the meanings of verbs. For example, the verb *jump* can be changed to the following forms: *jumped, jumping, jumps*. What is the name for these verb endings?

_____

b. Some verbs in a child's early sentences use all inflections. These verbs are called "pro-verbs." What are two common pro-verbs?

_____

c. The development of inflections in other verbs is driven by the temporal aspect of the verbs that a child is learning. Define each aspectual meaning listed below and identify the verb inflections used to create that aspect.

(1) Durative: _____

_____

(2) Momentary: _____

_____

17. a. The Wh-question words are learned in a specific order by children, no matter what language they speak. There is a group of early developing Wh-questions, and a group of later developing questions. Place the question words under their appropriate headings below.

Early Developing   **Late Developing**

_____   _____

_____   _____

_____   _____

_____   _____

b. Two factors determine this sequence of development of Wh-questions. Identify these two factors and describe how they separate the early from late developing question words.

(1) _____

_____

(2) _____

_____

18. a. Complex sentences are cumulative in that the meanings of the individual phrases build on each other to create a new meaning unique to the complex sentence. The chapter presents three types of meaning in complex sentences. List and define each type:

(1) _____

_____

(2) _____

_____

(3) _____

_____

b. These meanings can be expressed in two different forms. These forms are:

(1) _____

(2) _____

19.   The development of causal statements in children is significant because much of their interaction with their environment builds on their growing understanding of causal relations among members of their world. These language forms can often be difficult because they may require taking the perspective of another person. Bloom describes the order of development of causal language according to the child's ability to take another person's perspective. What are the steps of causal language development?

a. _____

b. _____

c. _____

20.   In order to converse with people in their environment, children must learn to share

the topic of discussion. The earliest form of topic sharing is _____ in which the child repeats what the adult says. Later, children start to add new information to a shared topic. These utterances with new information for a shared

topic are _____ productions.

21.   Bloom summarizes four major themes which are pervasive throughout the process of language development. These are important to remember when you study children and the language they use. What are the four themes?

a. _____

_____

b. _____

_____

c. _____

_____

d. _____

_____

ESSAY QUESTIONS

1. Children who are part of a deaf community in which sign language is used are exposed to sign as one language in their environment. How do you think the development of sign language would be the same as or different than the development of a spoken language in a child? Find references to support your view and briefly discuss the development of sign language as it compares to the development of spoken language.

2. According to the developmental perspective, language development takes place within the context of the overall growth of the child in all other facets of his or her life. The chapter contains many examples of how cognitive skills affect language development, but there are other interactions as well. Describe how you think each of the domains below could affect language development. How might a problem in one contribute to problems with language?

   a. Cognitive development:

   b. Social development:

   c. Emotional development:

   d. Motor skills/physical development:

3. One of the great debates is that of nature versus nurture. What are some traits children are born with that influence their language development (nature), and what are the factors from their environment that can affect development (nurture)? How might problems in one domain (nature) be compensated for by the other (nurture) or vice versa? Do you think our society places more value or resources on either nature or nurture? What leads you to your opinion?

4. Bloom mentions the work of Jean Piaget who studied the cognitive development of children. Piaget divides childhood into several stages of cognitive growth. Using outside references (developmental psychology textbooks are great), briefly describe the Piagetian stages of cognitive development that correspond to the period of language development presented in Bloom's chapter (ages 0–3 years).

5. The anthropological perspective on language development looks at language within the context of the social environment. Children must learn to use language according to the customs and practices of their respective cultures. One important skill to learn is how to address different people in the environment depending on their relationship to you. For example, if you needed someone to do you a favor, such as helping you locate a book you lost, think of how you would ask different people you know. Describe the words, voice quality, and overall manner you would use in asking the following people:

a. Your best friend:

b. Your parent:

c. A fellow student you have never met:

d. The head of your academic department:

e. Your younger sibling:

Give examples of how the social customs of your environment might be violated for any two of these people when you talk to them.

ACTIVITIES

1. Observation

Observe a child in the age range of 1–3 years old in any setting (at a day care center, in the park, at home, on video). First make notes about the following information:

Child's age: _____

Child's activity: _____

Child's communication partner(s): _____

Other pertinent information about the environment: _____

_____

Now write down 10 complete utterances the child says:

Analyze the 10 utterances in two ways:

a. Describe the form of each utterance according to the classifications presented in the box on page 197 in the chapter. What are the child's most typical forms of utterances?

b. Describe the communication purpose each utterance serves. Is the child requesting something, using a social routine, commenting on the topic, or using any other mental meaning or communication intent?

(1) _____

_____

(2) _____

_____

(3) _____

_____

(4) _____

_____

(5) _____

_____

(6) _____

_____

(7) _____

_____

(8) _____

_____

(9) _____

_____

(10) _____

_____

2. Timeline

On the following page there is a timeline ranging from the ages of 0–3 years. Several developmental hallmarks experienced by typically developing children are listed below. Mark these developmental milestones on the timeline. You may remember that many of these developments are described by a range of time over which the behaviors emerge instead of just one point in time. You may use either the range of time of development or the average age as a point in time, whichever you prefer. You will notice that some of the milestones listed below are from this chapter while others are not. You may need to consult outside references. Textbooks on child development are good resources. The purpose of including domains beyond language is to reinforce the developmental perspective that language emerges within the context of the overall development of the child.

Language

a. Communication through laughs, cries, and other nonverbal modes _____

_____

b. Babbling _____

c. First words _____

d. Vocabulary spurt _____

e. Simple sentences _____

f. Complex sentences _____

g. Negation expressed most often with single word "no" _____

h. Negation expressed through more complex forms _____

i. Causation expressed in complex sentences _____

j. Emergence of contingent conversation in which children add new information to

a shared topic _____

Cognition

a. Symbolic capacity _____

b. Piaget's sensorimotor stage of development _____

c. Piaget's preoperational stage of development _____

Motor

a. Begins to sit alone _____

b. Crawls successfully _____

c. Begins to walk _____

d. Has muscle control to begin potty training _____

Birth ←——→ 3 Years

Reference

Language Development by Robert E. Owens, Jr., Merrill Publishing Company, Columbus, OH. Copyright 1988 Merrill Publishing Company, Inc.

CHAPTER 6

Language Disorders in Children

LINDA SWISHER, Ph.D.

STUDY GUIDE

1. What are the differences between language disorders, such as aphasia, that are seen primarily in adults and developmental language disorders diagnosed in childhood?

    _____

    _____

    _____

    _____

2. Within what age range are developmental language disorders commonly diagnosed?

    _____

3. What are the three major categories of disorders discussed in this chapter for which developmental language impairments are primary features?

    a. _____

b. _____

c. _____

4. If children are identified at birth as being at risk for developmental language disorders, they can be closely monitored and treated throughout their early years. List four factors that indicate a child may be at risk for possible developmental language disorders:

   a. _____

   b. _____

   c. _____

   d. _____

5. Frequently children who appear to exhibit age-appropriate language skills during preschool later "grow into deficits." What is meant by "growing into deficits"?

   _____

   _____

   _____

   _____

   _____

6. During an evaluation for developmental language disorders, the speech-language pathologist must make three important decisions regarding the child's language skills. What are these three decisions?

   a. _____

   b. _____

   c. _____

7. To answer the three questions listed in exercise 6, the speech-language pathologist must measure three language components. Each component is defined below. Label each feature appropriately. Then, on the lines following each definition, briefly describe an example of how that component might be impaired in a developmental language disorder. Some examples can be found in the case histories at the end of Chapter 6 or in Chapter 5.

a. _____ : The variety of purposes to which language is put to communicate with other people including commenting, requesting, and regulating.

Example: _____

_____

b. _____ : The phonology, morphology, and syntax of language.

Example: _____

_____

c. _____ : The meanings expressed in language.

Example: _____

_____

_____

8. In order to make the decisions described in question 6 above, the speech-language pathologist must collect information about the child using a variety of techniques and resources. List five primary sources of information that the clinician might use:

a. _____

b. _____

c. _____

d. _____

e. _____

9. The speech-language pathologist will collect at least two types of data when assessing a child's language skills. The purposes of both measures are provided below. Identify the type of assessment procedure that fits each description.

a. _____ : Compares a child to age and socio-linguistic peers to corroborate existence of disorder.

b. _____ : Provides descriptive data regarding the nature of the disorder (language components affected) and how the child uses language (function).

10. Suppose that an evaluation by a speech-language pathologist reveals that a child is not hearing very well; or perhaps the clinician suspects delayed cognitive, motor, or social-emotional development. What must the speech-pathologist do before finalizing the diagnosis of a developmental language disorder?

_____

_____

11. a. What was the first law that required public schools to provide speech and language therapy to all school-aged children in need of them?

_____

b. When was this law passed?

_____

c. What does this law mandate?

_____

d. How was this law changed by P.L. 99-457 in 1990?

_____

_____

_____

e. What is meant by the term "least restrictive environment"?

_____

_____

_____

12. The author describes five principles that guide effective clinical practice. These principles are listed below. For each one, briefly describe the essential element of the principle that makes it important to clinical service.

a. Interdisciplinary approach:

_____

_____

_____

b. Provision of services in group and individual formats:

_____

_____

_____

c. Parent participation in intervention:

_____

_____

_____

d. Mainstreaming:

_____

_____

_____

e. Enhance functional skills in natural environments:

_____

13. Language disorders are key challenges faced by children with specific language impairments, mental retardation, and autism. Each of these conditions has a distinctive pattern of variables including the history, nature of the language disorder, and other co-existing disorders. To help you understand these three types of developmental language disorders, complete the profiles outlined below. Describe the child's level of function for each area of development. Add additional descriptive information that would be helpful to you. *Note:* It is important to remember that no two children with the same disorder will be exactly alike. Everyone is unique! The outline below is simply a way for you to organize some of the basic information about general patterns of language disorders.

Specific Language Impairment

Language (component): _____

_____

Intellect/Cognition: _____

_____

Other Handicapping Conditions: _____

_____

Etiologies/Historical Factors: _____

_____

_____

Age Disorder Is Noticed: _____

_____

Intervention Strategies: _____

_____

Additional Information: _____

_____

Mental Retardation

Language (component): _____

_____

Intellect/Cognition: _____

_____

Other Handicapping Conditions: _____

_____

Etiologies/Historical Factors: _____

_____

Age Disorder Is Noticed: _____

_____

Intervention Strategies: _____

_____

Additional Information: _____

_____

Autism

Language: _____

_____

Intellect/Cognition: _____

_____

Other Handicapping Conditions: _____

_____

Etiologies/Historical Factors: _____

_____

Age Disorder Is Noticed: _____

_____

Intervention Strategies: _____

_____

Additional Information: _____

_____

14. What is the relationship between a specific language impairment and a learning disability?

_____

_____

_____

_____

_____

ESSAYS

1. Take a moment to think about the impact that a developmental language disorder might have on the growth and development of a child. Discuss the potential impact of the disorder from the following perspectives: social, educational, and vocational. Provide one idea that might be used to improve the potential of the child in each of the three domains. These improvements might include services for the child or changes in the community.

2. The author(s) discuss the use of norm-referenced tests and behavioral observations as two key methods for gathering information about a child's language skills. For each of these two types of assessment tools, discuss three advantages and three disadvantages. How might the disadvantages be minimized to allow the best evaluation possible for the child?

3. The goal of any evaluation session is to maximize "representativeness." What does this term mean and how can it be achieved?

4. The public laws that mandate speech and language services in the public schools provide resources for treating children in the age range of birth to 3 years. What skills and factors are targeted for treatment during that time? Why do you think it is important to provide early intervention services for children at this young age?

5. The author(s) describe three different therapy approaches: child-oriented approaches, trainer-oriented approaches, and hybrid approaches. Discuss the key elements of each approach including details about the purpose of each, the populations for which each is appropriate, the materials and techniques, the settings, the goals, and the advantages and disadvantages.

ACTIVITIES

1. Ask your instructor to set aside some class time or a separate laboratory during which you can look over and try out some of the common tests used in analyzing the language skills of children. Pick three of these tests and sample some of the activities in each. For each of the tests, report the name, the purpose of the test, the population for whom it is appropriate, and your opinion about the test. What do you like or dislike and why?

2. The authors describe some of the adult language behaviors that either contribute to, or detract from, the development of language skills in children. Provide examples of at least three positive adult behaviors and three adult behaviors that are less supportive. Now, armed with this information, go out into your community to a park, shopping mall, zoo, or other setting where you can watch parents and children interact. Make a note of the occurrence of the adult behaviors listed above that you observe and the responses of the children. Based on these observations, can you identify the "growing edge" of the child's language? How might the parents change their behaviors to support the child's language development better?

   Notes: First, it is important to remember that parents *do not* cause language disorders. The purpose of this activity is simply to help you become aware that the way adults communicate with children can affect how the children use language in return. Second, you must be aware of the ethical aspects of "invasion of privacy." To guard against making unfamiliar parents nervous by observing them and their children, particularly if you are taking notes, you must first seek the permission of the parents prior to making an observation. Inform parents of what you want to do and why. Alternatively, you can simply make casual observations that you can write down later.

CHAPTER 7

Human Communication Disorders in Context and Environment

JAMES R. ANDREWS, Ph.D.

STUDY GUIDE

1.   When conducting therapy, speech pathologists and audiologists must consider factors such as the people involved in therapy, the setting or place therapy is conducted, and the materials and techniques utilized. Describe each of these three factors as they have been applied in the traditional service delivery model.

People: _____

_____

Place: _____

_____

Techniques: _____

_____

2. In recent years, a new service delivery model has emerged that focuses on providing therapy in the context of the client's life. Describe the same three variables as they might be applied in contextual therapy.

People: _____

_____

Place: _____

_____

Techniques: _____

_____

3. This chapter presents two main paradigms which form the basis for models of clinical practice. One paradigm is the linear cause-effect paradigm which forms the basis for the medical model. Describe seven assumptions of the medical model that form the foundation of the linear paradigm:

a. _____

_____

b. _____

_____

c. _____

_____

d. _____

_____

e. _____

_____

f. _____

_____

g. _____

_____

4. The second service delivery model is the systemic paradigm. Describe the seven assumptions that form the foundation of the systemic perspective on treatment.

a. _____

_____

b. _____

_____

c. _____

_____

d. _____

_____

e. _____

_____

f. _____

_____

g. _____

_____

5. Each of the following statements represents either the linear or systemic paradigm. Read each and label with an 'L' if it typifies the linear paradigm, or with an 'S' for the systemic paradigm.

a. ____ Phenomena are not studied in their natural environment

b. ____ Based on cause-effect relationships

c. ____ Depicted as circular interactions among contextual participants

d. ____ Each individual's perception of truth is accepted as valid

e. ____ Reduces a problem to independent, individual components

f. ____ Each communication event is unique in relation to its context

g. ____ Problems are related to the experience of the system as a whole

h. ____ Challenging as a new perspective for professionals and clients

i. ____ Traditional thought pattern of Western civilization

6. In the systemic paradigm, the unit of treatment includes the client, the clinician, and any family members, friends, professionals, or other persons who are significant in the client's daily environment. This group of people is referred to as:

_____

7. **a.** As suggested above, the definition of the treatment system will vary depending on the paradigm selected by the clinician. For each of the two paradigms, describe who is expected to change their behavior in response to intervention based on their inclusion in the treatment system.

Linear: _____

_____

Systemic: _____

_____

b. In what setting or at what time is change expected to emerge for each of these treatment systems?

Linear: _____

_____

Systemic: _____

_____

8. The role of the clinician differs in each treatment system as well. Describe the function of the clinician in each of the paradigms:

Linear: _____

_____

Systemic: _____

_____

9. Finally, the two treatment systems vary in terms of their utilization of counseling techniques. Describe how clinicians using each of the two paradigms would incorporate counseling into their intervention.

Linear: _____

_____

Systemic: _____

_____

10. The four systemic principles that relate to treatment in context are listed below. They are followed by four statements that describe the systemic principles as they might be applied to speech pathologists. Match each principle with its correct description based on information in the text.

   A. One part of a system cannot be understood in isolation from the rest of the system.

   B. Change in one part of the system creates change in other parts of the system.

   C. Transactional patterns of the family determine the behavior of family members.

   D. A family's structure, organization, and developmental stage are important factors in determining the behavior of family members.

Now identify each description of a principle:

_____ Every interactive system has a set of both spoken and unspoken values, attitudes, and assumptions which are like traditions that exert significant influences on the behavior and communication of members in the system.

_____ Family members can communicate more information among themselves than is apparent to outsiders based on their mutual interactive system. Thus, the communication behavior of one member of the system is more complete when it is analyzed in the context of the entire system.

_____ Each system has a hierarchy with each member fulfilling certain roles and responsibilities. The identity and abilities of each person within the system must be respected in providing therapeutic recommendations.

_____ Family members can either enhance or diminish the effectiveness of treatment because of interactions in which new behaviors of the client cause new reactions in other members of the system. These reactions are likely to influence the direction the client takes the new behavior.

11. The third systemic principle states that patterns of attitudes, beliefs, and actions shared by members of the system exert a considerable influence on the behaviors and changes in behaviors of members. In the columns below, provide some examples of both overt and covert communication patterns and values that you feel might influence your treatment program. Some examples in the text will get you started, then see if you can think up some more, possibly from your own experience.

Overt   **Covert**

_____   _____

_____   _____

_____   _____

_____   _____

_____   _____

12. In the case example for the third systemic principle, which focuses on transactional patterns, the author stresses the importance of positive successful communication with a child regardless of the medium (such as gesture replacing speech). Why do you think it is so important to encourage the child's communication in any positive way instead of focusing entirely on speech?

_____

_____

_____

_____

_____

13. In discussing the fourth systemic principle of system organization, the author describes developmental stages that are important to consider because they contribute to the values and resources in a system. Provide three examples of different developmental stages for a family and describe how the values and resources might affect a treatment plan:

a. _____

_____

_____

_____

b. _____

_____

_____

c. _____

_____

_____

_____

14. The text provides three examples of contextual therapy in professional practice with communication disorders. These examples demonstrate the interaction of many important people in the client's environment. What are the three examples of contextual therapy listed in the chapter?

a. _____

b. _____

c. _____

15. a. Public Law 99-457 organized intervention services targeting children in the age range from birth to 3 years of age. These family-centered services are based on the foundation of the following three principles described in the text:

(1) _____

(2) _____

(3) _____

b. Can you identify five advantages of this focus on family responsibility in intervention? Consider the effects on the family, child, and community in terms of social, educational, vocational, and financial health.

(1) _____

_____

(2) _____

_____

(3) _____

_____

(4) _____

_____

(5) _____

_____

16. In the chapter, the author cautions clinicians that the systemic treatment design will lead to clinician involvement in interactive systems that may vary greatly in their organization, values, orientations, and social customs. Clinicians need to be able to provide treatment without being judgmental of a system that is different from their own. Below are some examples of clients with whom you may or may not be able to identify. For each one, discuss issues that you might find challenging, even though you would be open to treating each one as a speech pathologist or audiologist. If none of these clients are thought-provoking for you, provide an example of a client who would provide challenges for you in terms of entering a system unfamiliar to you.

a. A child on your caseload was born with fetal alcohol syndrome. The birth mother, who drank during pregnancy, is attempting to participate in programs to reduce her substance abuse and to learn parenting skills while she raises her daughter. Provide your reaction:

_____

_____

_____

_____

b. A young adult on your hospital rehabilitation ward has communication disorders resulting from a head injury received in a motorcycle accident. The accident occurred while the man was trespassing illegally in an area off limits to motorcycles because of the extremely dangerous terrain. The man was not wearing a helmet at the time of the accident. Provide your reaction:

_____

_____

_____

_____

c. A woman in your clinic has undergone a medical change in gender from male to female. As part of adopting the female identity, she would like to work on her voice and speech characteristics to make them more feminine, and she would like to join the transgender therapy group sponsored by your clinic for this purpose. Provide your reaction:

_____

_____

_____

_____

d. If you have any other examples of a client who would challenge you in terms of presenting an interactive system notably different from your own, please share that in the space below:

_____

_____

_____

_____

17. If the clinician is to successfully facilitate change in an interactive system, the clinician must be accepted into the system. What is the term from the field of family therapy that refers to this acceptance of the clinician into the system?

_____

18. What are some of the ways in which a clinician can promote acceptance into the system?

a. _____

_____

b. _____

_____

c. _____

_____

d. _____

_____

19. What does the term "co-evolution" mean?

_____

_____

_____

_____

_____

20. How do you know if co-evolution is an outgrowth of successful treatment?

_____

_____

_____

_____

_____

21. According to the author, co-evolution should occur in a nonhierarchical manner. How might the development of a hierarchy in the system be a detriment to the growth and change of the system? Provide three possible reasons or problems?

a. _____

_____

b. _____

_____

c. _____

_____

22. Although speech-language pathologists and audiologists do not provide counseling beyond that directly related to issues of communication skill, clinicians do use counseling techniques to facilitate the growth of interactive systems. What are some purposes for which counseling techniques are useful?

a. _____

b. _____

c. _____

d. _____

e. _____

23. The author lists several counseling techniques that are useful. Select three of these from the text and define them:

a. _____

b. _____

c. _____

24. The author suggests that intervention is most successful when the therapeutic techniques and suggestions are offered in a format that is consistent with many patterns and characteristics already present in the interactive system. Thus, the clinician is not causing upheaval of the system, but is introducing new behaviors so that they can easily be incorporated into the existing format of the system. What is the term that describes this respect for the existing form of the system?

_____

ESSAY QUESTIONS

1. In many ways the systemic paradigm seems a lot "looser" than the linear paradigm because in the systemic paradigm no predetermined structure, truths, or requirements are imposed strictly by the clinician. To a certain degree, the clinician has to "go with the flow" of a system already in existence. However, this does not mean that the systemic paradigm advocates therapy programs that are disorganized and nonproductive. Somehow, the clinician must keep in mind an agenda of goals and therapeutic techniques that might be appropriate. In a short essay answer, describe some of the challenges that might be faced by a clinician in trying to organize and guide therapy along a systemic paradigm so that the clinician can exert professional influence without becoming clearly dominant as in the linear paradigm. How might some of these challenges be managed successfully?

2. According to the author, the perspective and professional beliefs of the clinician determine his or her approach to treatment. As a clinician, do think you would prefer working in a linear paradigm or a systemic paradigm? Why? Which do you think would be better for your clients? Which might be easier for you as a clinician to conduct? Do you think you would always pick one or the other, or might you try combinations of the two? Why?

3. The author states that, although speech-language pathologists and audiologists use many counseling techniques, they are not professional counselors. The boundary of professional counseling needs to be clearly respected. This may be difficult in a systemic paradigm in which many issues in the system may affect your intervention for communication disorders, and some of these issues may be beyond your professional qualifications. How do you decide where to draw the boundaries in terms of topics you can address and those that you should not?

Use this example: You are treating a preschool child for stuttering. As you begin to interact in the family system you discover that there are problems in the marital relations of the parents that are creating a stressful home environment. Often the parents are not as supportive of their child's efforts to communicate as you would like them to be, and you suspect that the tension created by their relationship problems contributes to decreased quality of the child's communication environment. How might you deal with this situation so that you could promote better parental communication styles with their child? What variables can you address within your professional domain and qualifications and which can you not treat? What would you do about topics that you recognize as areas of concern but are not qualified to treat?

ACTIVITIES

1. Pick a system of which you are a member. This may include your family, friends or living companions, a group at school, or your job setting. Define at least three or four members of the system; the roles and functions of each member; the underlying assumptions, values, and beliefs of the system; the overt behavior patterns characteristic of the system; and the manner in which the system solves problems. Can you identify a problem within the system? How might you approach it from a systemic point of view?

2. Learn to recognize just how much information can be gained from the context beyond verbal communication. This will help you recognize all of the different types of information that contribute to the communication environment so that you will be better able to identify these variables when providing treatment to a system. Select a favorite T.V. show, preferably one with which you are familiar. Watch an episode with the volume turned off. If you are able to, tape the show so that you can watch it later with the volume on to evaluate the accuracy of your interpretations without the sound. Describe as much as you can of the plot of the show. How did you know this? Include examples of different mediums of information you used to understand the show such as props on the show and the gestures and mannerisms of characters. Were you able to understand the humor if it was a comedy? How much did you rely on your previous experience with the show to interpret this episode? How adequate

do you feel all these forms of context were in replacing verbal communication? If you taped the show, watch it again with the volume on and describe any changes in your interpretations.

3. Pretend that you are a speech-language pathologist who will be evaluating the communication skills of a 3-year-old boy whose parents are concerned about his speech and language development. Think about the context of your evaluation session and the variables that you need to consider when preparing for the session. What variables beyond his verbal skills do you think would affect the performance of the child? How might you prepare for this from a systemic point of view to ensure that you are able to evaluate the child to the best of your potential? Some examples to get you started include the setting and the materials that you use. Provide more detail on these and other factors you can think of.

Neurological Bases of Communication Disorders

RAY D. KENT, Ph.D.

STUDY GUIDE

The Neuron

1. In the space below, draw a diagram of a typical neuron. Label the **dendrites,** the **cell body,** the **axon,** and the area(s) at which the neuron **synapses** with other neurons. Indicate the direction in which the nerve impulse travels down the neuron.

2.   **a.** How does information travel along a neuron?

_____

     b. How is this information transmitted to successive neurons?

_____

3.   What is the neurological role of myelin?

_____

_____

_____

4.   What is the microscopic space across which neurotransmitters travel to propagate the nerve impulse?

_____

5.   The term "nucleus" has two distinctly different meanings in the field of neuroanatomy. Define the two different structures.

     a. _____

_____

     b. _____

_____

6.   What is the difference between a nucleus (the macroscopic type) and a ganglion?

_____

_____

7.   **a.** What is a bundle of axons in the central nervous system called?

_____

b. What are they called in the peripheral nervous system?

_____

8.   **a.** What are the two types of neurons presented in the text?

_____

b. What are the functional differences between the two types?

_____

_____

_____

_____

_____

The Human Nervous System

9.   What is the functional relationship between the central nervous system (CNS) and the peripheral nervous system (PNS)?

_____

_____

_____

_____

_____

10. On the brain diagram below, label the following structures and landmarks:

a. Which hemisphere is this?
b. The four primary lobes
c. The central and lateral fissures
d. Broca's area
e. Wernicke's area

f. The brainstem
g. Primary Motor Cortex (Motor Strip)
h. Primary Sensory Cortex
i. Primary Auditory Cortex
j. The cerebellum

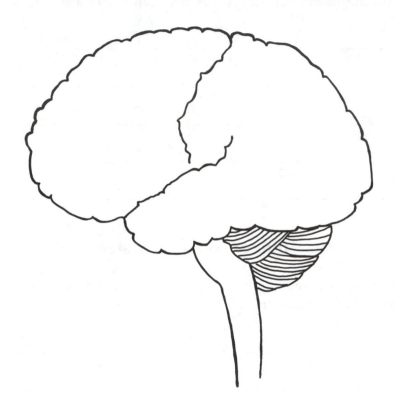

11. What is the name of the "bark-like" outer surface of the brain?

_____

12. What aspect of the surface of the brain allows for a greater number of neurons than would otherwise be expected?

_____

_____

_____

_____

13.   **a.** What structure allows for communication between the two hemispheres of the brain?

_____

   b. What is this structure composed of?

_____

_____

14.   What structure in the brain is often referred to as the sensory "way station" of the cerebrum?

_____

Where would sensory information most likely go from here?

_____

_____

_____

15.   Motor neuron pathways beginning in the right hemisphere innervate the

_____ side of the body.

   a. What is the neurological term for this phenomenon?

_____

   b. How does this occur?

_____

_____

_____

16.   New brain imaging techniques seem to be popping up every few months. (By the time this text gets to you, other methods may have arrived on the scene to provide physicians and clinicians with increasingly accurate pictures of the brain's structures and activities.) Although the techniques involved in many of these procedures are quite complex, it is useful to know at least what type of information the images are presenting. Below, match the diagnostic information desired with the most applicable current imaging technique(s).

_____ **a.** Brain structure after a recent head injury

_____ **b.** Electrical activity in an area of the brain during a particular function

_____ **c.** Oxygen and/or glucose usage in an area of the brain during a particular function

_____ **d.** Determining whether a stroke-afflicted area has significant cell death

1. PET
2. MRI
3. EEG
4. CT

Language and the Brain

17. What functions do the following lobes perform with respect to speech, language, and hearing?

a. Frontal Lobe: _____

_____

b. Parietal Lobe: _____

_____

c. Temporal Lobe: _____

_____

d. Occipital Lobe: _____

_____

18. Language production and comprehension in the brain is not carried out by one particular group of cells (unless, of course, you consider the entire brain as such). Rather, different aspects of language are carried out in separate yet connected areas (how separate and how connected are topics of much debate in the field of neuroscience.) The text mentions two important areas of language function in the brain. What are these two areas, and what functions are they thought to perform?

a.

_____

_____

b.

_____

_____

19. How are these areas and connected within the brain?

_____

20. In what hemisphere are these language areas found in the majority of humans?

_____

Are all aspects of speech and language found in this hemisphere?

_____

Of what neurological phenomenon is this an example?

_____

21. Motor control for speech is extremely complicated and very important. Many structures in the brain are set up to help plan, initialize, and regulate speech mechanism control. List the five primary structures involved in the motor speech production process, as mentioned in the text. Briefly describe the general role that each plays during speech production.

a.

_____

_____

b.

_____

_____

c.

_____

_____

d.

_____

e.

_____

_____

_____

22. **a.** What pathway describes the primary route that neuronal information takes from the primary motor cortex to muscles?

_____

b. Which pathway connects the motor-regulating structures to this primary pathway?

_____

23. Less obvious than direct motor control of speech is the sensory information required to accurately and efficiently run the speech machine. List four particular anatomical structures about which the brain would need information for speech control.

_____

_____

_____

24. Identify the most likely category of communicative disorders that could result from damage to the following areas:

a. Broca's area   _____

b. Primary auditory cortex   _____

c. Basal nuclei   _____

d. Primary motor strip (orofacial area)   _____

e. Wernicke's area   _____

f. Pyramidal pathway   _____

ESSAY QUESTIONS

1. Discuss the role of the central nervous system in the organization and control of motor behavior during speech production.

2. The composite motor behavior required for speech production may involve movements in different parts of the body at the same time (e.g., lips, tongue, larynx, and respiratory system). How are these movements regulated by the CNS?

3. Sometimes it is necessary to sequence the movement in a single structure over time. How are movements by the same structure sequenced over time? Is sequential movement of a structure dependent on the central nervous system, the peripheral nervous system, or both?

4. Many neurogenic communication disorders fall under the two general categories of aphasias and dysarthrias. What are the primary differences between these two disorders?

5. The concept of language localization in the brain is a subject of great controversy among neuroscientists. Answers to some of the questions raised above are by no means agreed on by all neuroscientists, but they are generally accepted by many due to their usefulness in correlating certain symptoms with particular areas of brain damage. Briefly describe the three currently prevailing theories on the localization of language in the brain:

   a. Centers and Pathways Model
   b. Convergence Zone Model
   c. Modular Model

ACTIVITIES

1. After you have gone to a dentist for work on your teeth, write down how it feels to have your mouth "deadened." (If you have not been to a dentist lately, talk with someone who has.) Were any of the muscles or structures used for speech production affected by the anesthesia? How did it impair your ability to produce speech? Write down your observations. Be specific.

2. Interview a person who has a neurologically based communication disorder. Determine how the neurological problem has interfered with normal communication. How does the patient feel about the nature of the communication disorder?

3. While talking, try to imagine where the tip of your tongue or where the tongue body is positioned during each speech sound produced. Say the vowels "ee, ah, oo, uhh." Can you feel where your tongue is? Now say the consonants "d, t, k, g, s, and th." Could you do a better job of determining where your tongue was during the production of those consonants? Why?

4. If your instructor can provide a delayed feedback device, try speaking with zero delay in the sound that reaches your ear and compare how that feels with a condition where you delay the speech by 200–250 msec. What differences did you observe? Were you able to speak as well with delayed auditory feedback? Why?

5. Observe videotapes of a person with aphasia and a person with dysarthria. What differences did you observe in their manner of communication?

6. Compare the relative difficulty of listening to a conversation in a crowded room when your eyes are open, as compared to listening in a crowded room with your eyes closed. What differences did you observe?

7. With your index finger, tap your finger on a table as many times per second as you can. Now, using all four fingers on your hand, sequence the finger taps in a "finger rolling" or "finger drumming" maneuver. Were you able to tap faster with more than one finger involved? Why? What does this activity tell us about motor control?

Neurogenic Disorders of Communication

LEONARD L. LaPOINTE, Ph.D.

STUDY GUIDE

Vocabulary

Define the following terms.

1. a. Neuropathology:

_____

_____

b. Categories of neuropathology include (list and define):

_____

_____

_____

_____

_____

_____

2. Cerebrovascular accident:

_____

3. Necrosis:

_____

4. Dementia:

_____

_____

_____

5. Aphasia:

_____

_____

6. Verbal Paraphasias:

_____

_____

7. Neologisms:

_____

_____

8. Alexia:

_____

9. Agraphia:

_____

10. Emotional Lability:

_____

_____

11.　Contre coup:

_____

_____

12.　Pragmatics:

_____

_____

13.　Dysarthrias:

_____

_____

_____

_____

14.　Apraxia of Speech:

_____

_____

_____

15.　Dysphagia:

_____

16.　Aspiration:

_____

17.　Modified Barium Swallow:

_____

18.　Prosody:

_____

_____

Concepts

1. During a stroke, blood flow to the brain can be disrupted in two ways. What are they?

   a. _____ : Excessive bleeding such as a blood vessel in the brain bursting.

   b. _____ : Stationary or moving blood clots that block the flow of blood to the brain.

2. What is the critical duration of a stroke after which permanent damage is caused to brain cells?

   _____

3. Aphasia results in the impairment in the ability of the patient to use two primary domains of language, semantics and syntax. Define each below.

   a. Semantics: _____

   _____

   _____

   b. Syntax: _____

   _____

   _____

4. Four primary modalities of language use are affected by aphasia. Although some modalities may be more affected than others, depending on the location and severity of the brain damage, impairments are typically seen in all four. List the four modalities of language use below:

   a. _____

   b. _____

   c. _____

   d. _____

5. The severity of a communication disorder caused by neuropathology may depend on many different variables. However, the three primary contributors to the severity of disorder are:

a. _____

b. _____

c. _____

6. As discussed in the chapter, a wide variety of linguistic behaviors is observed in patients with aphasia. However, many of these behaviors can be grouped into clusters to create different aphasia "syndromes" that result when particular regions of the brain suffer damage. The primary distinction in describing aphasia is between the fluent and nonfluent categories. However, within each of these categories there are several types of aphasia that differ slightly from each other. The following exercise is designed to help you review the language behaviors you might see in patients with a particular type of aphasia.

The names of the different aphasia types are presented below. Below each type, the lesion site and behaviors you would want to observe are listed. On the blank line, describe the lesion site and how each behavior would appear to you in a patient. An example is provided for you. The starred item (*) under each type highlights the behavior essential for differentiating that particular type of aphasia from the others. Pay special attention to this feature.

Nonfluent Aphasias

	Broca's	Transcortical Motor	Global
Lesion:	_____	_____	_____
Production:	_____	_____	_____
Comprehension:	_____	better than production	* _____
Naming:	_____	_____	_____
Repetition:	_____	* _____	_____
Self-Monitor:	_____	_____	* _____

Fluent Aphasias

	Wernicke's	Transcortical Sensory
Lesion:	_____	_____
Production:	_____	_____
Comprehension:	_____	_____
Naming:	_____	_____
Repetition:	_____	*_____
Self-Monitor:	Poor ability to detect errors	_____

	Anomic	Conduction
Lesion:	_____	_____
Production:	_____	_____
Comprehension:	_____	_____
Naming:	*_____	_____
Repetition:	_____	*_____
Self-Monitor:	_____	_____

7. The author points out that the brain damage which causes many of the language, communication, and behavior deficits also causes changes in the physical appearance and function of the patient. List three physical problems commonly experienced by victims of brain injury. For each of the three problems, give an example of how this disability might affect their daily life experiences.

a. _____

_____

_____

b. _____

_____

c. _____

_____

_____

_____

8. On page 375 in the chapter, LaPointe presents a table listing many of the behaviors observed in patients with right hemisphere impairment. In the box on page 373, LaPointe also provides a case study of a patient who has right hemisphere impairment. Read the case study and write down seven behaviors that are symptoms of the injury. Then select from the table on page 375 the category and name of the deficit demonstrated by each behavior. An example is provided below:

Example: Patient reports that he loses track of the main idea during long conversations. This behavior is an illustration of a linguistic deficit of poor auditory comprehension for lengthy, complex material.

a. _____

_____

_____

_____

b. _____

_____

_____

c. _____

_____

_____

_____

d. _____

_____

_____

_____

e. _____

_____

_____

_____

f. _____

_____

_____

_____

g. _____

_____

_____

_____

9. a. Dementia is a condition of progressive intellectual decline. The most common symptom of dementia is:

_____

However, dementia is characterized by deterioration in other intellectual capacities including:

_____

_____

b. Describe how each of these contributes to communication disorders in persons with dementia. Review the section on communication and dementia for examples.

_____

_____

_____

_____

_____

_____

_____

10. The most common cause of dementia, accounting for 50% of all cases, is:

_____

11. There are two general classes of neuromotor speech disorders. They are:

_____

12. Differentiate neuromotor speech disorders from neurogenic language disorders. What are the different communication functions impaired by each?

_____

_____

_____

_____

_____

REMEMBER THAT BOTH NEUROMOTOR SPEECH AND NEUROGENIC LANGUAGE DISORDERS CAN—AND OFTEN DO—OCCUR TOGETHER IN THE SAME PERSON.

13. There are five aspects of the speech production process that could be impaired due to dysarthria. List the five aspects:

a. _____

b. _____

c. _____

d. _____

e. _____

14. Compare the symptoms of dysarthria with those of apraxia of speech.

Dysarthria	**Apraxia of Speech**
_____	_____
_____	_____
_____	_____
_____	_____
_____	_____
_____	_____
_____	_____

15. Some of the movements of our bodies are automatic, somewhat similar to the automaticity of reflexes. Automatic movements include those that are often part of basic life support. Other movements are purposeful movements that require planning in the motor association cortex of the brain. (*Note:* purposeful movements do not have to be planned consciously.) Dysarthria impairs both automatic and planned movement because the muscles are always weak and/or uncoordinated due to damage anywhere along the neuromuscular system. In apraxia, automatic movements are preserved but purposeful movements are compromised because of the person's inability to plan and program those movements in the brain. Apraxia is a general term referring to the inability to program and move parts of the body in a planned, purposeful manner despite the absence of any paralysis or weakness. Based on this definition, provide description and examples of each of the following two forms of apraxia. Compare the two. What type of movement might be preserved and what type of movement might be impaired for each? Think of examples of movements you need each day. Samples are contained in the text of the chapter.

a. Oral apraxia:

_____

_____

b. Apraxia of speech:

_____

_____

16. Dysphagia occurs most frequently with what communication disorder discussed in the chapter?

_____

17. Why do speech disorders and swallowing disorders commonly co-exist?

_____

_____

_____

18. Dysphagia can be a very serious threat to a patient's health and life for two reasons. What are these reasons?

a. _____

_____

_____

b. _____

_____

_____

19. List five possible symptoms of dysphagia:

a. _____

b. _____

c. _____

d. _____

e. _____

20. Why might the following members of a medical team all participate in treating a patient with dysphagia?

a. Physician: _____

_____

b. Speech pathologist: _____

_____

c. Occupational therapist: _____

_____

d. Radiologist: _____

_____

e. Dietician: _____

_____

f. Nurse: _____

g. Other: _____

21. Speech-language pathologists must read the medical charts of patients in the hospital to determine what medical issues might affect the communication of patients and the efforts of clinicians to help them. These charts are sometimes hard to read and it's not because the doctor's have illegible handwriting! All medical professionals use many abbreviations of common terms to make their writing faster and easier. Many of the terms you learned in this chapter have abbreviations that you will see in medical charts. Can you figure these out?

a. CVA = _____

b. TBI = _____

c. AOS = _____

d. PET = _____

e. RHI = _____

f. CHI = _____

g. PTA = _____

h. DAT = _____

ESSAY QUESTIONS

1. You tested a patient who suffered a CVA to the left side of his brain to see how well he understands language. When you read the patient's file, you noticed that he needs to wear a hearing aid because he has a hearing loss, but he did not have the hearing aid with him in the hospital during the test. What problems might you encounter when you try to test how well he understands what you say? What is the difference between deficits in auditory comprehension and deficits in auditory acuity? How might each affect the results you see on the test? How might you determine which problem a patient has if you had no prior information? How might deficits in auditory acuity influence auditory comprehension? Address these questions in a short paragraph.

_____

_____

_____

_____

_____

_____

_____

_____

_____

Now draw a parallel between this situation and the similar example of visual acuity versus visual perception in reading comprehension. What is the difference between visual acuity and perception? How might this influence both the things you do to test a patient and how you analyze the results?

_____

_____

_____

_____

_____

_____

_____

_____

_____

2. As LaPointe emphasizes several times, the patients you see with communication disorders are all individuals with their own values, life styles, and abilities. Each patient is unique and must be appreciated for his or her individuality. Therefore, brain injury will impact each person differently.

Assume you have two patients who have each suffered brain injuries of similar types and severities. The injury was a TBI resulting in mild-to-moderate right hemisphere impairment. While these women should be able to return to functional activity and possibly even regain employment, they are facing many of the challenges discussed for RHI. Biographical data for each patient are presented below:

Patient A: 52-year-old female; Education — Ph.D.; Occupation — college professor in literature; Social — married with no children. Husband reports patient tends to be withdrawn and lives quiet life style with hobbies such as reading that do not require much social interaction. Patient and husband have always been happy with more secluded life.

Patient B: 32-year-old female; Occupation — day care attendant; Education—high school graduate; Social — divorced with sole custody of two children, ages 6 and 10 years. Patient has good social support network of friends and relatives and is active in social functions such as going to movies (comedies) and going out with friends. Family reports patient was occasionally slightly depressed prior to injury because of financial and emotional pressures of being a single parent.

Describe how the various physical, psychological, educational, vocational, and social factors presented above might affect how each of these patients might cope with the brain injury, the degree to which the patients might return to the activities of their previous life styles, and the adjustments that might have to be made for new life styles. What challenges might pose specific problems for each? What tools does each possess to help her adjust? Feel free to make up more information about the patients if it helps you develop your rationale for defining strengths and challenges.

STUDENT WORKBOOK FOR INTRODUCTION TO COMMUNICATION SCIENCES AND DISORDERS

3. LaPointe mentions that one consequence common to RHI is left:

_____

Research the definition of neglect. How does it compare to visual acuity? What behaviors might be seen in a patient with neglect? Can you think of any ways to help that patient compensate for neglect? What might you teach them?

_____

_____

_____

_____

_____

_____

_____

4. a. In discussing TBI, LaPointe introduces the comparison between **focal lesions** and **diffuse brain damage**. What is the difference between the two in terms of type of lesion as well as nature, extent, and prognosis of impairments seen in patients?

_____

_____

_____

_____

_____

_____

b. In a related manner, define and compare **stable** versus **degenerative** conditions. Can you provide an example of each? How might each affect your ideas about patients' prognoses and how to help them?

_____

_____

_____

_____

_____

_____

_____

_____

5. Patients with brain injury often do not fully recover all functions so they are not as independent as they were prior to the injury. Residual deficits are usually present. LaPointe suggests that, when patients cannot recover or adequately relearn behaviors, the environment must often compensate for the patient and provide support to help the patient function successfully. The environment can include anything or anybody with which the patient interacts.

You have a right-handed patient who suffered a severe CVA to the left frontal lobe. She suffers from nonfluent aphasia with coexisting dysarthria, changes in personality so that her behavior is different than it was prior to the insult, and significant weakness in the right side of her body that impairs mobility and the use of her right hand.

What are some ways that the environment could compensate for functional deficits in this patient? What adjustments might have to be made in her physical environment (house) and social environment (family and friends) to help her to participate functionally and gain as much independence as possible? Below are several categories of issues in which environmental manipulations might be warranted. What solutions can you suggest?

a. Difficulty writing due to weakness in right hand: _____

_____

_____

_____

b. Difficulty communicating due to complications from nonfluent aphasia and unintelligible speech from dysarthria even though she often knows what she wants to tell someone:

_____

_____

_____

_____

_____

c. Occasional discomfort of friends who have not been around the patient since her stroke and are taken off guard by her behavior which is not characteristic of how she acted prior to the stroke:

_____

_____

_____

_____

_____

d. Difficulty getting around her house because of physical limitations caused by weakness on the right side of her body:

_____

_____

_____

_____

e. Hypothesize about another challenge she might face and how the environment could be manipulated to help her cope:

_____

_____

_____

_____

_____

ACTIVITIES

1. LaPointe states that some of the most troubling types of neurogenic communication disorders come in the form of impairments in understanding the subtleties in language use such as figures of speech and humor. These people may be able to follow the literal meaning of language, and they may be able to perform daily tasks with verbal instruction. However, they may miss the richer meaning of language and be robbed of satisfactory communication with their environment because of their impaired abilities for abstract interpretation of linguistic and nonlinguistic cues that occur during communication.

   Our environment, especially the media, is peppered with this abstract use of language as well as communication through nonverbal modes. Your assignment is to attempt to appreciate just how much subtle yet significant meaning such patients might miss in communication because of their deficits in comprehending the abstract linguistic and nonlinguistic information in a setting.

   Pick a favorite situation comedy on T.V. As you watch it, write down 10 examples of the humor in the show. Include both language humor (jokes) and situation humor (slapstick). Describe the subtleties of communication such as double meanings of what people say or meanings conveyed through body language that might be confused with the literal interpretations of what the characters say.

   Reviewing the chapter, especially the description of RHI, describe how much of the show a patient who watched it might have had difficulty understanding or the misinterpretations that might have occurred due to the humor, use of language in general, or the nonlinguistic behavior of characters that communicated meaning.

a. _____

b. _____

c. _____

d. _____

e. _____

f. _____

g. _____

h. _____

i. _____

j. _____

2. Observation of a brain-injured patient: Your instructor will provide an opportunity for you to observe a patient with a neurogenic communication disorder either through a video tape or direct observation in a clinical setting. Describe the following characteristics about the patient:

a. Background (provided by instructor): _____

_____

_____

_____

_____

b. Physical symptoms of brain damage: _____

_____

_____

_____

_____

c. What problems does the patient have in understanding language?

_____

_____

_____

_____

d. What problems does the patient have in expressing her- or himself through language?

_____

_____

_____

_____

_____

e. What problems does the patient have in his or her speech?

_____

_____

_____

_____

_____

f. Does the patient demonstrate any behavior that seems unusual and might be attributed to the brain damage? Describe:

_____

_____

_____

_____

_____

g. What problems does the patient have in reading or writing?

_____

_____

_____

_____

h. Do you see any environmental compensation occurring (e.g., people helping the patient succeed at a task)?

_____

_____

_____

_____

i. What are the greatest challenges you think this patient faces in functioning in the community?

_____

_____

_____

_____

j. Any other observations you feel are important:

_____

_____

_____

_____

_____

Scientific Substrates of Speech Production

KENNETH N. STEVENS, Ph.D.

STUDY GUIDE

Sound Sources and Filters

1. The airway extending from the larynx to the lips may be identified as the

    _____

2. The structures that can move and affect the shape of the vocal tract during speech

    production are called:

    _____

3. In the spaces below name seven different articulators that may be used during
    speech production.

    a. _____

    b. _____

    c. _____

d. _____

e. _____

f. _____

g. _____

4.   What is the primary function of the respiratory system during speech production?

_____

_____

_____

_____

5.   The theory of sound production discussed in this chapter is the:

_____

6.   When air is flowing smoothly in laminar flow (flow without turbulence), as during normal breathing, is sound produced?

_____

7.   Name two ways that the airstream is converted into sound during speech production.

a. _____

_____

_____

b. _____

_____

_____

8. The pitch of the sound produced by vocal-fold vibration within the larynx is determined by:

_____

_____

_____

9. The spectrum of the fluctuating airflow through the glottis resulting from vocal fold vibration (laryngeal tone or glottal sound source) is made up of:

_____

_____

_____

10. In the space below draw the spectrum of a normal glottal sound source.

11. True "whispering" does not contain any speech segments that are voiced (i.e., no periodic changes in airflow produced by the vocal folds). Still, we can perceptually differentiate whispered vowels and other whispered speech sounds. We can even tell the difference between "voiced" and "voiceless" sounds during whispered speech production. What is the sound source for vowels during whispering?

_____

_____

_____

_____

_____

12. With respect to the position of the vocal folds shown in Figure 10–4 of the text, what would be the position of the vocal folds during whisper?

_____

_____

13. We can still hear a "pitchiness" to the sounds produced during whisper. (*Note:* you cannot have a true pitch without a periodic sound source like that produced by vocal-fold vibration.) What accounts for the fact that some whispered sounds are perceived as higher or lower than others?

_____

_____

_____

_____

_____

_____

_____

14. If the glottal spectrum is held constant during the production of various vowel sounds, what causes the differences in the vowel qualities (i.e., what causes the vowel /i/ to sound different from the vowel /ae/)?

_____

_____

_____

_____

_____

_____

_____

_____

_____

15. The filtering characteristics of the vocal tract vary greatly from person to person. Children have small vocal tracts and adults have larger vocal tracts. Will the size of the vocal tract influence what frequencies will be resonated by that "filter"? In what way?

_____

_____

16. In the United States (or in any other country with a variety of dialects), we can often denote a sound pattern or a "sound quality" that is characteristic of a certain region of the country. What variables in the general shape or usage of the vocal tract can lead to regional differences in vocal resonance?

_____

_____

_____

_____

17. In an even more striking instance, blood relatives often have similar sounding voices due to the similarities of their vocal tract characteristics (think of the Kennedys, for example). What anatomical variables, besides length of the vocal tract, could influence its filtering characteristics (and could be transferred from one generation to the next genetically)?

_____

_____

_____

_____

Waveforms and Spectra

18. a. A sinusoidal waveform (or combinations of them with frequencies that are multiples of a fundamental frequency) can be used to describe any phenomenon (heat, light, sound) that repeats itself systematically over time (i.e., is periodic). What variation is typically displayed in a sound waveform that reaches the ear of a listener?

_____

b. List some other objects or events from your experience whose motion or variation might be depicted in a sinusoidal waveform. Include cases that may require "ideal" conditions (e.g., no friction). Draw a waveform for one of them, indicating the "frequency," "amplitude," and "period" of your object's motion.

_____

_____

19. Shown below is a waveform.

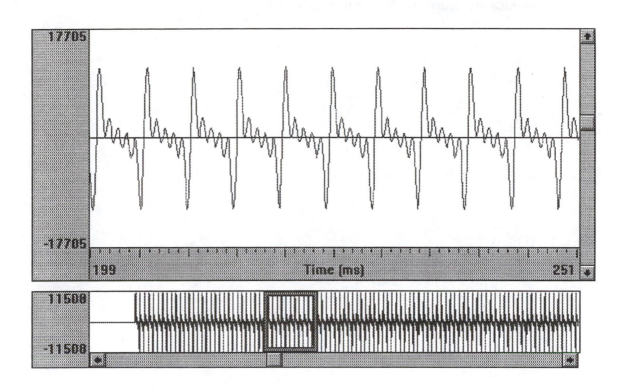

a. What type of waveform is it?

_____

b. How is it different from a sinusoidal waveform?

_____

_____

_____

c. What is the period of the waveform? _____

d. What is its fundamental frequency (F_0)? _____

e. List the frequencies of the first five harmonics of the waveform.

_____

f. Below, sketch a line spectrum of the waveform shown in question 19 above, including just the first 5 harmonics. Assume that the amplitudes of the harmonics decrease as the frequency increases.

20. Assume that a female vocal tract is 15 cm in length. If we assume that the velocity of sound is 35,400 cm/sec, what would be the first three formant frequencies for a uniform vocal tract of that length?

_____

21. If the fundamental frequency of the female identified in question 20 is 250 Hz, what harmonics (and their frequencies) are nearest to the three formants shown above and would receive most amplification?

_____

Speech Acoustics

22. a. Refer to Figure 10–9 in the textbook. In what direction does the first formant move when a speaker shifts the vowel from /i/ in "beet" to the vowel /ae/ in "bat"?

_____

b. How does the tongue position in the oral cavity change when this shift is made?

_____

23. a. What area(s) of the vocal tract are changed the most when changing from the vowel /i/ as in "beet" to the vowel /u/ as in "boot"?

_____

b. What articulatory movements are required to achieve this change?

_____

_____

_____

24. What would you expect to happen to the value of the second formant in a vowel like /a/ if it were produced with lip rounding?

_____

25. a. The stop consonants /t/ and /k/ are produced at different places of articulation within the vocal tract. What is acoustically similar between these two sounds?

_____

_____

_____

_____

_____

b. How do these two sounds differ, and what causes the difference?

_____

_____

_____

_____

_____

_____

ESSAY QUESTIONS

1. What is the source-filter theory of speech production? What are the basic assumptions of this theory? Include comments about how this theory might be useful in describing differences between normal speech production and speech produced by someone with a pathology of the speech production apparatus.

2. What are the differences between source spectra for voiced sounds and for voiceless sounds? Why do these differences occur?

3. What is the difference between a spectrum and a spectrogram? Define each of these terms. Sketch an example of each.

4. Discuss the concept of the bandwidth of a filter. Compare a filter that passes a narrow band of frequencies with one that passes a wide band of frequencies. What are the implications of filter bandwidth for our knowledge of speech acoustics?

5. Based on what you have learned from this chapter, speculate on how formant transitions (formant trajectories) during speech production are related to the timing of articulatory movements within the vocal tract?

ACTIVITIES

1. Glass bottles provide us with an excellent demonstration of sound sources and filters. Fill a glass bottle (12–16 oz works well) three-quarters full with water. Blow over the top of the bottle to produce a tone.

   a. What is acting as the sound source?

   _____

   _____

   _____

   _____

   b. What is acting as the acoustic filter?

   _____

   _____

c. Listen to the pitch of the sound produced when you blow across the opening and cause the air column in the bottle to resonate. What would you expect to happen to the pitch of the sound if you drained water from the bottle? Why?

_____

_____

_____

_____

Carry out the experiment to verify your predictions.

2. Produce a sentence in your normal voice. Now, produce the same sentence in a whisper. Did they sound alike? Could you distinguish all of the same sounds? Could you tell the difference between voiced and voiceless sounds even during whisper? How could you do that?

3. Listen carefully and also monitor your articulatory movements as you produce the following words and phrases: "I, pity pat, aurora, mean, moon, toot, we were away, cupcake, sizzle." Make careful notes about what you heard. Were all of the sounds the same length? Did they have different pitches? Were they all voiced? How did the tongue body move? Was the soft palate lowered at any time during the utterance?

CHAPTER 11

Genetics, Syndrome Delineation, and Communicative Impairment

ROBERT J. SHPRINTZEN, PH.D.

STUDY GUIDE

1. The author introduces four main disciplines in this chapter. Although there are close relations among these disciplines, each discipline should be recognized for its own focus of study. Define and differentiate the following:

    Dysmorphology: _____

    _____

    Syndromology: _____

    _____

    Human Genetics: _____

    _____

    Molecular Genetics: _____

    _____

2. Congenital anomalies occur in what percent of the population?

_____

3. The anomalies described in this chapter are deviations from either normal structure or normal function. Provide three examples of each from the chapter:

Structure: _____

Function: _____

4. a. The term used to refer to abnormal embryonic and fetal development is:

_____

b. What is the difference between the embryo and the fetus?

_____

_____

5. In the discipline of dysmorphology, the word *syndrome* means a pattern of multiple anomalies in a single individual. To be classified as a syndrome, this pattern must meet three requirements which are:

a. _____

b. _____

c. _____

6. a. What does the acronym DNA stand for: _____

b. What does DNA do in our bodies? _____

_____

7. a. There are two branches in the study of human genetics: clinical genetics and molecular genetics. Define each branch:

Clinical genetics: _____

_____

Molecular genetics: _____

_____

b. The study of genetics produces two profiles of information about each patient. These are the phenotype and the genotype. Define each profile and identify the branch of genetic study listed above that generates it:

Phenotype: _____

_____

Genotype: _____

_____

8. a. There are four different categories of identifiable causes, or etiologies, for anomalies. These are defined below. Name each cause:

(1) _____ : Exposure by the mother to agents such as alcohol or radiation that enter the embryo's environment and interfere with the embryo's development.

(2) _____ : Abnormal alteration, or mutation, of a single gene.

(3) _____ : Anomalies caused by forces redirecting or inhibiting the growth of the embryo, or by forces that tear or mutilate the embryo.

(4) _____ : Broad spectrum of anomalies caused by abnormalities in the long strands of DNA that carry the genetic material.

b. There are also two categories of unknown genesis syndromes whose etiologies are unidentifiable. Label the definitions of these two:

(1) _____ : Anomaly patterns that have been seen before in other people, yet all individuals are unrelated in terms of their karyotypes, history of teratogenic exposure, and family heredity so no consistent etiology can be defined.

(2) _____ : Anomaly patterns that have not been seen or reported before in any other person.

c. Give two reasons why it is important to identify the etiologies of syndromes, if possible:

(1) _____

(2) _____

9. What are chromosomes?

_____

_____

Each human cell contains how many chromosomes? _____

These are organized into how many identical pairs? _____

The last pair of chromosomes in each cell, which may or may not be identical,

determines what characteristic of the embryo? _____

An analysis of the chromosomes is called a _____

10. Provide four types of chromosomal abnormalities that may cause anomalies:

a. _____

b. _____

c. _____

d. _____

11. a. Although many anomalies may accompany chromosomal abnormalities, what two categories of anomalies may be of particular concern for development of speech, language, and hearing?

(1) _____

(2) _____

b. What other anomalies are also strong indicators of chromosomal abnormalities?

(1) _____

(2) _____

(3) _____

12. **a.** Chromosomes are long strands made of DNA. DNA consists of small segments of material which are the units of human heredity. These units are called:

_____

b. The genes are arranged along each chromosome in a specific order, and this arrangement serves as the instructions for the developing embryo. The name for this arrangement of genes and the information it provides is:

_____

c. An alteration in the structure or order of this arrangement might cause anomalies. Such an alteration is called a:

_____

13. **a.** Just as chromosomes are paired, the genes on each chromosome also have identical pairs on the corresponding chromosome (except for the chromosomes to determine sex). The embryo inherits one gene in each pair from each parent. It is important to know that genes are paired because the inheritance of mutant genes varies depending on which genes in an inherited pair are mutated. Label the three patterns of inheritance which may cause anomalies:

(1) _____ : Both members of the gene pair are mutant. Inheritance risk is 25%.

(2) _____ : One member of the gene pair is mutant. Inheritance risk is 50%.

(3) _____ : Mutant gene carried on the X chromosome with traits more commonly expressed in boys who have only one X chromosome than in girls who usually have a normal X chromosome to offset the abnormal one.

b. There are two other patterns of genetic mutation which do not fit into the inheritance patterns defined above. Describe these other two patterns:

(1) Multifactorial: _____

_____

(2) Contiguous: _____

_____

14. a. The author describes five categories of teratogenic influences that interfere with the environment of the developing embryo. In the spaces provided, name each of the five categories and provide three examples of members of each category:

Teratogenic Category   **Examples**

(1) _____   _____

_____

_____

(2) _____   _____

_____

_____

(3) _____   _____

_____

_____

(4) _____   _____

_____

_____

(5) _____   _____

_____

_____

b. Why is it difficult to predict the effects of teratogenic influences on an embryo?

_____

_____

_____

_____

15. In mechanically induced syndromes, the development of the embryo would have proceeded normally except for the influence of mechanical forces which interrupt normal development. Define the two types of mechanical forces and provide one example of each:

a. Disruptions: _____

Example: _____

_____

b. Deformations: _____

Example: _____

_____

16. Multiple anomalies may be the result of either a syndrome or a sequence. Differentiate the two by labeling each definition appropriately:

a. _____ : Multiple anomalies which all originate out of one common cause and co-occur in a fairly consistent, recognizable pattern.

b. _____ : A single malformation or deformation that may have many possible causes, and in turn leads to other secondary anomalies as the baby develops.

17. **a.** Syndromes affecting hearing may cause anomalies in any of the four divisions of the ear: outer, middle, inner, and neural. List two examples of anomalies in each division:

Outer: _____

Middle: _____

Inner: _____

Neural: _____

b. Anomalies of the outer ear are often associated with anomalies of the _____

ear, but are not commonly associated with anomalies of the _____ ear.

18. Language impairment should be suspected in any syndrome which presents with any of the following three findings:

a. _____

b. _____

c. _____

19. Why is the brain particularly susceptible to damage from malformation, metabolic disturbances, or teratogenic influences?

_____

_____

20. Articulation disorders often accompany syndromes with oral anomalies. For each of the oral anomalies listed below, describe how you think each might impair the ability of a child to articulate speech sounds:

a. Dental abnormalities:

_____

_____

_____

_____

b. Tongue abnormalities:

_____

_____

_____

_____

c. Neurologic impairment:

_____

_____

_____

_____

21. Children with anomalies in the oral cavity, such as cleft palate, may use atypical articulatory substitutions such as glottal stops to compensate for speech sounds such as oral stops that they are not able to produce. Using information about the oral anomalies in cleft palate and compensatory glottal stops in the text and glossary, explain why oral stops are difficult for children with cleft palate and how glottal stops might be a logical compensatory strategy.

_____

_____

_____

_____

_____

_____

_____

_____

22. List four possible types of laryngeal anomalies present in syndromes which may contribute to voice disorders:

a. _____

b. _____

c. _____

d. _____

23. Not all voice disorders are part of a syndrome. In considering the potential for a voice disorder to be related to a syndrome, it is very important to first examine the child's voice history and patterns of voice use to determine if the voice disorder might be a form of what common occurrence in children:

_____

24. Resonance disorders may take three main forms. Label each resonance disorder defined below:

a. _____ : Too little nasal resonance due to small nasopharynx, nasal cavity, or insufficient opening to the nasal cavity.

b. _____ : Muffled oral resonance quality caused by abnormalities in the size or shape of the oral or pharyngeal cavities.

c. _____ : Too much nasal resonance due to insufficient separation between the oral and nasal cavities.

25. Because diagnosis of syndromes is often a long and complicated process, speech-language pathologists and audiologists should be aware of warning signs of syndromes in their patients so that the clinicians can make appropriate referrals when warranted. The following three signs would warn the clinician that the patient should be examined by a qualified professional for the potential of a syndrome:

a. _____

b. _____

c. _____

ESSAY QUESTIONS

1. At the beginning of the chapter the author discusses how the term "genetics" has replaced the term "birth defects" in the professional language. Why did this change occur? Other terms have also undergone evolution. For example, children today are often referred to as "developmentally delayed" instead of "retarded" as used to be the case. Can you think of any other examples of evolutions of terms in the medical field or in society in general? What might cause these changes in terms? Why is it important for speech-language pathologists and audiologists keep abreast of these changes?

_____

_____

_____

_____

_____

_____

2. Correct identification of syndromes and sequences is extremely important to ensure proper care and treatment of a child with multiple anomalies. The author presents several areas of knowledge that contribute to the identification and treatment of a syndrome. These topics are the phenotypic spectrum, the natural history, and the prognosis. Discuss each of these three topic areas including the information they provide about the syndrome and how this information is used by health care providers and families in the proper treatment of children with syndromes.

a. _____

_____

_____

b. _____

_____

_____

c. _____

_____

3. According to the author, many syndromes can be treated so that, even though a child may not have normal structure or function, he or she can still live a relatively long and productive life. However, there are some syndromes that have very poor prognoses either because of their degenerative nature or because effective treatments have not yet been found. There is a question as to the wisdom and ethics of providing treatments for these patients when the treatments carry little or no advantages. Discuss your opinion on this situation. What variables might you consider when thinking about treatments for cases with poor prognoses? These include the nature of the disorder, the nature of the treatment, the philosophy of the clinician, and the concerns of the family, and the care and comfort of the patient. What other factors might you consider? Provide general arguments to support your opinion about this issue.

4. In the case report at the end of the chapter, the author mentions the low Apgar score which warned doctors immediately after the baby's birth that there might be a problem. Research the Apgar scale and discuss its purpose, organization, and the information it provides.

ACTIVITIES

This chapter presents many different syndromes and sequences as examples. The following exercise is designed to help you organize a reference source that you can use for quick information about some of the syndromes. While only a few syndromes are assigned here, you might want to use this format to research additional syndromes which you find affect the speech, language, and hearing in children.

1. Velo-cardio-facial (Shprintzen) Syndrome

Etiology: _____

Category of etiology: _____

Phenotypic spectrum: _____

_____

_____

Natural history: _____

_____

Prognosis: _____

_____

Implications for speech: _____

_____

Implications for language: _____

_____

Implications for hearing: _____

_____

Other: _____

2. Stickler Syndrome

Etiology: _____

Category of etiology: _____

Phenotypic spectrum: _____

_____

_____

Natural history: _____

_____

_____

Prognosis: _____

_____

Implications for speech: _____

_____

Implications for language: _____

Implications for hearing: _____

_____

_____

Other: _____

3. Now select one syndrome from the chapter or a syndrome that is of particular interest for you from a different source and outline its features using the format below:

Syndrome: _____

Etiology: _____

Category of etiology: _____

Phenotypic spectrum: _____

Natural history: _____

Prognosis: _____

Implications for speech: _____

Implications for language: _____

Implications for hearing: _____

Other: _____

CHAPTER   12

Voice Disorders

LORRAINE OLSON RAMIG, Ph.D.

STUDY GUIDE

1.   What is another word that means the same thing as "phonation"?

   _____

2.   Your voice is produced by what part of the anatomy that is often referred to as your "voice box?"

   _____

3.   The larynx is constructed out of three cartilages. Match the name of each cartilage to its description below:

   _____   Thyroid cartilage

   _____   Cricoid cartilage

   _____   Arytenoid cartilages

   A. Pair of small pyramidal cartilages that sit on top of the back of the cricoid cartilage.

   B. Largest cartilage in the larynx forming the front and side walls of the larynx.

   C. Ring of cartilage below the thyroid cartilage.

4.   These three cartilages form a frame. Inside of this frame are two "folds" of tissue that can open, close, and vibrate to produce voice. What are these "folds" of tissue called?

   _____

5. In addition to cartilages, the larynx also has five sets of muscles that we use to control and change our voices. Fill in the following chart with the points of attachment for each muscle, the physiologic changes caused when each muscle contracts, and the changes created in how you perceive or hear the voice. Some examples have been provided for you.

Hints: The points of attachment are simply the names of the cartilages to which each muscle is attached. The muscle is named after the cartilages to which it is attached. Remember that each muscle comes in pairs — one on each side of the body!

Muscles	Points of Attachment	Physiologic Changes	Perceptual Changes
Thyroarytenoid	Example: Thyroid cartilage Arytenoid cartilage		
Cricothyroid		Example: Stretches and thins vocal folds	
Lateral cricoarytenoids			
Interarytenoids			Example: Produce voice and increase loudness
Posterior cricoarytenoid			

6.   **a.** When vocal folds open or move apart, we say they:

_____

       b. This opens the path from the mouth and throat above to the lungs below. What is the main purpose for opening the vocal folds that allows us to live?

_____

7.   **a.** When the vocal folds close, or move together, we say they:

_____

       b. This closes the path from the mouth and throat to the lungs. Can you think of two reasons why we need to close our vocal folds? _Hint:_ One is very important when we eat.

       (1) _____

       (2) _____

8. In order to produce voice, the adducted vocal folds must be acted upon by some force which would cause them to vibrate. This force does not come from the larynx itself, but from some other part of the body. What is the power supply that causes the vocal folds to vibrate?

_____

9. As we breathe out, the airstream going through the adducted vocal folds causes the folds to vibrate (continuously open and close). During vibration, the vocal folds act like a valve on the exhaled airstream causing bursts of energy that form an acoustic sound wave above the vocal folds. We hear this sound wave as:

_____

10. The respiratory system that provides the power supply for vocal fold vibration consists of the lungs, rib cage, and abdomen. Name two muscles that are used to control the respiratory system:

_____

11. As the airstream rushes out of the lungs toward the vocal folds, it passes through the windpipe. Another name for windpipe is:

_____

12. a. If you could look at a cross-section of the vocal folds, you would see five layers of tissue. Name the five layers starting with the outermost layer and moving to the innermost:

(1) _____

(2) _____

(3) _____

(4) _____

(5) _____

b. Which layer vibrates most during phonation?

_____

13. The following statement is false. Correct it to make it true:

"The glottis is the space between the vocal folds when they are adducted."

Correction: _____

_____

14. Which cranial nerve innervates the larynx? Provide both its name and number.

Name: _____

Number: _____

15. a. The rate of vocal fold vibration is calculated as the number of vibrations per second. The term used to refer to this rate of vibration is:

_____

b. How fast do the vocal folds of males and females typically vibrate?

Males: _____

Females: _____

c. Why this difference between males and females?

_____

_____

_____

16. The sound that comes out your mouth is not the same sound that was produced by your larynx. Why?

_____

_____

_____

17. As with many communication disorders, the diagnosis and treatment of voice disorders is often the product of input from professionals representing many different disciplines. The following five professionals work with patients with voice disorders. Match each professional with the description of his or her contribution to care of the patient with voice disorder:

_____ Otolaryngologist	**A.** Diagnose and treat medical conditions of the ear, nose, and throat.
_____ Neurologist	**B.** Work with vocal performers such as singers and actors; use artistic techniques to enhance the voice.
_____ Psychologist	**C.** Diagnose and treat medical conditions of the nervous system that affect the larynx.
_____ Vocal coach	**D.** Diagnose and treat emotional problems that impact health and use of the voice.
_____ Speech (voice) pathologist	**E.** Diagnose and treat disorders of voice of medical, psychological, or use/abuse origin.

18. One goal in the assessment of voice disorders is to establish a relationship between how the voice sounds (perceptual characteristics), and what the larynx and vocal tract are doing to create that sound (physiology). Below are descriptions of the three primary physiologic behaviors of the larynx. Identify the perceptual characteristic that accompany each.

_____ : The degree of vocal fold adduction and subglottal air pressure determines the sound pressure level of the acoustic signal.

_____: Vocal fold adduction, vibratory stability, and other vocal tract characteristics determine the tone of the voice.

_____: The length and tension of the vocal folds determine the fundamental frequency.

19. Although there are many ways of describing voice qualities, the author describes some of the most common perceptual terms for voice quality. List three examples of perceptual voice qualities:

a. _____

b. _____

c. _____

20. Voice quality can be affected by parts of the vocal tract other than the larynx. One example is the nasal quality of the voice which is determined in part by the amount of the acoustic signal that is allowed to enter and resonate in the nasal cavity.

Excessive nasality is called: _____

Insufficient nasality is called: _____

21. Why do you think hyponasality is common when you get a cold?

_____

_____

_____

22. The author lists two ingredients that are necessary in a healthy voice to produce the best quality of acoustic signal. What are these two ingredients?

a. _____

b. _____

23. The author illustrates some commom changes that occur in people's voices as they age. As an example, describe below the phenomena of the voice change typically experienced by teenage males. Why do their voices change so much? How is the physiology of the larynx changing? What perceptual qualities does this create?

_____

_____

_____

_____

24. Another term for a voice disorder is:

_____

25. The communication impairment resulting from a disordered voice depends on the following two variables:

a. _____

b. _____

26. There are three major etiological categories of voice disorders. List the three main types of causes:

a. _____

b. _____

c. _____

27. a. What is the definition of vocal misuse/abuse?

_____

_____

b. The author provides eight examples of life-style habits or behaviors that constitute vocal misuse/abuse. List all eight.

(1) _____

(2) _____

(3) _____

(4) _____

(5) _____

(6) _____

(7) _____

(8) _____

28. List five perceptual examples of poor voice quality that are the result of vocal misuse/abuse:

a. _____

b. _____

c. _____

d. _____

e. _____

29. Three physiologic changes may result from vocal misuse/abuse. Label each below:

_____ : Blisters on the vocal folds.

_____ : Ulcerations caused by vocal hyperfunction and/or gastro-esophageal reflux.

_____ : Callouses that form at the point of maximal vocal fold collision.

30. In psychogenic voice disorders, the larynx is usually capable of producing a normal voice, but the disordered or extreme emotions of the individual prevent a normal voice production. For each example of psychogenic voice disorder listed below, briefly describe the cause and the perceptual evidence:

Musculoskeletal Tension Disorder:

Cause: _____

Perception: _____

Conversion Voice Disorder:

Cause: _____

_____

Perception: _____

_____

_____

Mutational Falsetto:

Cause: _____

Perception: _____

_____

31. As referred to in the name, psychogenic voice disorders often include both vocal and psychological/emotional components. What do you think is the role of the speech-language pathologist in diagnosing and treating each of these components? What other professionals might become involved?

_____

_____

_____

_____

32. The medical/physical conditions that may cause voice disorders are many and varied. Below, list the six categories of medical/physical disorders and one example from each. Some examples are provided for you:

Etiology	Example
a. _____	Dystonia
b. _____	Fractured cartilages
c. _____	Laryngeal web
d. _____	Hypothyroidism
e. _____	Papillomata
f. _____	Laryngeal cancer

33. Following surgical removal of the larynx (laryngectomy) for laryngeal cancer, the patient must find a new "voice" source to allow him or her to continue to communicate effectively through speech. Two alternatives are described below. Identify each:

Electrolarynx: _____

_____

_____

_____

Esophageal Speech: _____

_____

_____

_____

34. Assessment of voice disorders may involve many types of measurements to gain insight into how the larynx is working. List six types of information that may be obtained in an assessment of voice.

a. _____

b. _____

c. _____

d. _____

e. _____

f. _____

35. Disorders of the nervous system may affect the larynx and result in a voice disorder. List three neurological disorders that may affect voice production.

a. _____

b. _____

c. _____

36. Treatment of voice disorders may involve any combination of approaches that is appropriate for each individual patient. The author lists four categories of common treatment approaches. What are they?

a. _____

b. _____

c. _____

d. _____

ESSAY QUESTIONS

1. Why is a medical examination of the larynx by an otolaryngologist necessary prior to beginning voice therapy?

Compare and contrast medical intervention such as surgery or pharmacological treatment and behavioral voice therapy. When should each be used? Should one be considered before the other and why? In discussing each, remember to address the overall health and well-being of the individual beyond the voice disorder. Provide examples of at least one voice disorder that warrants medical treatment and one indicating voice therapy.

2. The author discusses a continuum of voice quality ranging from breathy—normal—pressed/harsh. Describe each of these three points along the continuum. Discuss each of these voice qualities in terms of the physiology that creates the quality, the acoustic characteristics, the perceptual characteristics, and whether that quality is considered disordered or not.

3. Although voice disorders are serious concerns for every patient, the impact of the disorder on an individual's quality of life may depend on many variables. Can you think of some variables that might influence each person's adjustment to the disorder? Discuss five variables. (*Hint:* These might include resources to help the person cope as well as demands placed on the individual.)

Now let's discuss a specific example. Suppose that similar hyperfunctional voice disorders are diagnosed in a professional singer and in a retired farmer. What might the impact and concerns be for each person? How might you, as the SLP, approach treatment for each? Consider the variables you discussed above.

4. Review the author's discussion in the text of primary and secondary etiologies, and the example of having a cold. What are the definitions of primary and secondary etiologies? Discuss each using another example: vocal misuse/abuse and vocal nodules.

How might a cycle be formed in which the primary and secondary etiologies feed on each other? How could this cycle best be broken to restore a healthy voice?

ACTIVITIES

1. Observe how different emotions are conveyed through the voice. Select three examples of different emotions expressed in the voice that you observe in your daily interactions with people or on radio or television. For each example, describe the following:

    a. The perceptual characteristics
    b. The information/expression conveyed
    c. The physiologic functions of the larynx that you think created this voice
    d. Whether you think this is an example of healthy or unhealthy use of the voice

2. Select two voices that you have heard in your environment, on radio, or on television. One voice should be very pleasing and appealing to you, while the second should be a voice that you do not like. Describe both the pleasing and annoying voices including the following details:

    a. Pitch
    b. Loudness
    c. Voice quality
    d. Why you do or do not like the voice.
    e. How the voice affects your perception of the person/character as a whole.
    f. Whether you think the unpleasant voice is truly disordered or just annoying to you.
    g. Any other pertinent details or opinions about each voice.

3. Review the discussion of vocal misuse/abuse with its examples in the text. Now select a person whom you see frequently and keep a log of his or her vocal abuse/misuse over several days (you may even keep a log on your own voice). Describe each behavior that is harmful and keep track of the number of times you observe that behavior. At the end of the observation period, use your data to answer these questions:

    a. What was your subject's vocal hygiene like in terms of the type and amount of vocal use and misuse?
    b. In your opinion, do you feel your subject is at risk for a voice disorder based on the vocal habits that you observed?
    c. What advice might you give this person to help him or her improve vocal hygiene or address a possible voice problem?

CHAPTER 13

Fluency and Stuttering

DAVID PRINS, Ph.D.

STUDY GUIDE

1.   What is meant by the term fluency?

   _____

   _____

2.   How is stuttering related to fluency?

   _____

   _____

3.   What two components make up the stuttering event?

   a. _____

   b. _____

4.   List three core features that can occur during a stuttering event:

   a. _____

   b. _____

   c. _____

5.   Whose speech may contain core disfluencies?

_____

6.   With regard to stuttering, what produces accessory features?

_____

7.   Name three aspects of a client's stuttering episodes that are observed and measured when attempting to determine the severity of stuttering?

a. _____

b. _____

c. _____

8.   On the continua shown below, descriptively label the ranges of behavior expected for each parameter identified in answer #7 above. (Provide descriptors at the ends of each continuum to indicate what "mild" to "severe" quantities, or conditions, would exist at these extremes.)

←——————————————————————————————→

_____   _____

←——————————————————————————————→

_____   _____

←——————————————————————————————→

_____   _____

9.   How is the severity of stuttering events related to the degree of handicap associated with the disorder?

_____

_____

_____

10. Why is the term "intermittent" applied to stuttering?

_____

_____

11. List five or more conditions that can reduce or eliminate stuttering.

a. _____

b. _____

c. _____

d. _____

e. _____

f. _____

g. _____

12. During what period of linguistic development is normal disfluency prevalent in most children?

_____

_____

_____

13. What problem does the "overlap phenomenon" present to the clinician attempting to determine whether or not a child is an early stutterer?

_____

_____

_____

_____

14. What three features of preschool children's disfluent speech are analyzed to help differentiate between early stuttering and normal disfluency? How do they differ between these two cases?

a. _____

_____

_____

b. _____

_____

_____

c. _____

_____

_____

15. What types of situations are often associated with disfluency and signs of early stuttering?

_____

16. How did Van Riper's description of stuttering development in 1971 differ from Bloodstein's?

_____

_____

_____

17. What do Van Riper's and Bloodstein's reports tell us about the nature of stuttering development?

_____

_____

_____

18.   What is meant by the prevalence, versus the incidence, of stuttering?

_____

_____

_____

19.   Is the prevalence of stuttering consistent across cultures?

_____

_____

20.   When we ask, "What causes stuttering?" what features of the disorders are we usually trying to explain?

_____

_____

_____

ESSAY QUESTIONS

1. Even the most eloquent speakers are disfluent on occasion. Describe a disfluency experience you have had. What were the characteristics of your speech? Describe the situation you were in and how you felt during (and perhaps after) the episode.

2. The author points out an important distinction between the terms "disability" and "handicap of stuttering." How would you distinguish these terms? Give an example of how the terms might be used in describing someone who stutters chronically.

3. Briefly describe the four phases in the development of stuttering as put forth by Bloodstein.

I. _____

_____

_____

II. _____

_____

_____

III. _____

_____

_____

IV. _____

_____

_____

4. What evidence exists for a genetic link to stuttering? Why does it appear that a genetic source is neither necessary nor sufficient to account for stuttering?

_____

_____

_____

_____

_____

_____

_____

5. Develop a table to show various theories of the causes of stuttering. For each, include its period of ascendancy, the category of approach it takes to stuttering, its major proponent(s), and a brief summary of its main points regarding the cause and treatment of stuttering.

ACTIVITIES

1. Carefully observe the speech and language patterns of three children who are between 2 and 4 years of age. Keep a log of the number and types of disfluencies evident in their speech.

2. Describe what it feels like to speak in front of a large audience. Are those feelings much different from the way a stutterer must feel? Explain your answer.

3. Make a tape recording of one of your casual conversations with a friend or family member. Listen to the recording and transcribe exactly what you hear. Is normal speech characterized by the use of complete sentences? Did you observe any disfluencies? What were they? Describe what you learned from this experience.

4. Visit a speech clinic and observe a clinical therapy session with a client who stutters. (Preferably, the observations should be made through a one-way mirror so as not to disturb the therapy session. If no such facility is available, ask your instructor how you might complete this activity.) Describe what types of stuttering behavior were exhibited by the client. What did the clinician do to help the client?

5. For a period of not less than 1 week, take time to talk to an acquaintance who is shy or who does not communicate easily in most public settings. Honestly *care* about what that person is doing, or is feeling. Did the person's behavior change during the period of time that you have taken special time to care about, and talk to, the person? How did it change? Why do you think the person's behavior changed as it did?

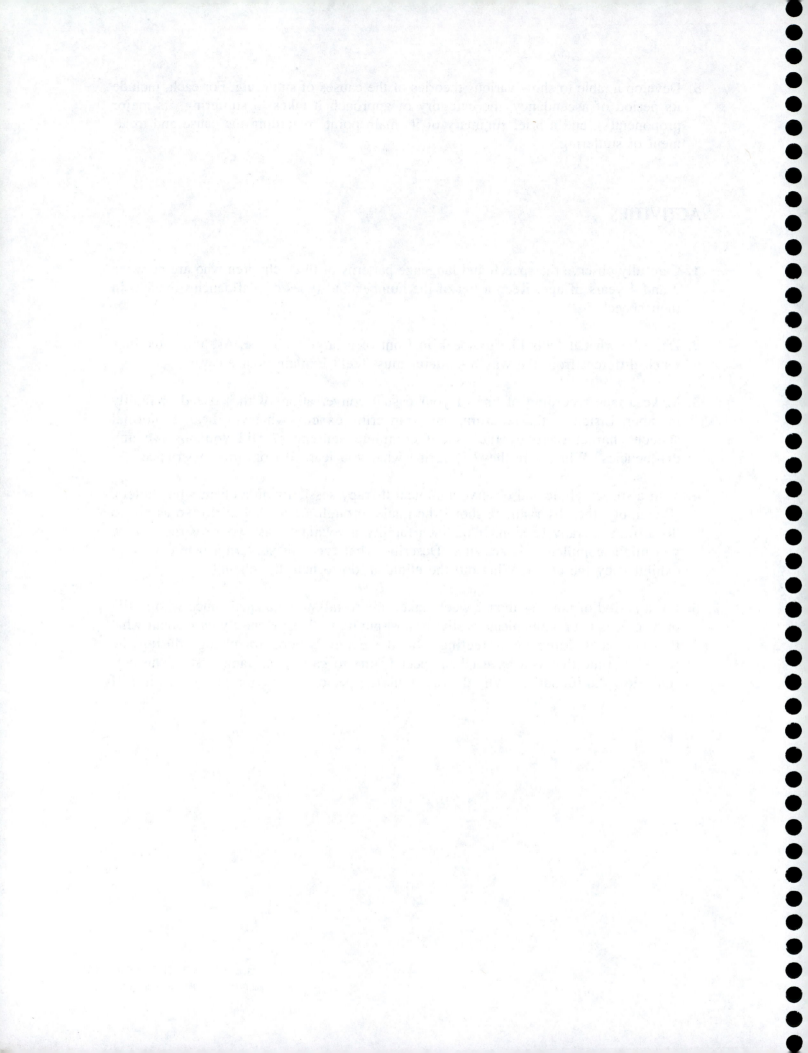

Sound Information: Scientific Substrates of Hearing

CHARLES I. BERLIN, Ph.D.

STUDY GUIDE

1.   What are the three major divisions of the human ear?

     _____

2.   What two structures make up the outer ear?

     _____

     _____

3. What functions do the outer ears of humans serve?

   a. _____

   b. _____

4. Name the structure that forms the boundary between the outer ear and the middle ear? What is its primary function?

   _____

   _____

5. a. The three bones of the middle ear are collectively known as:

   _____

   b. List the name of each bone, in order from the eardrum to the boundary of the inner ear.

   (1) _____

   (2) _____

   (3) _____

6. What is the function of the bones of the middle ear?

   _____

7. a. The tube that connects the middle ear to the nasopharynx is called the:

   _____

   b. What purpose does it serve?

   _____

8. a. The portion of the inner ear dedicated to the hearing sense is called the:

   _____

   b. What sense does the remaining portion contribute to?

   _____

9. On the diagram below, label the structures referred to in questions 1–8.

a. Outer ear   **g.** Ossicles

b. Middle ear   **h.** Malleus

c. Inner ear   **i.** Incus

d. Pinna (auricle)   **j.** Stapes

e. External auditory canal   **k.** Cochlea

f. Eardrum (tympanic membrane)

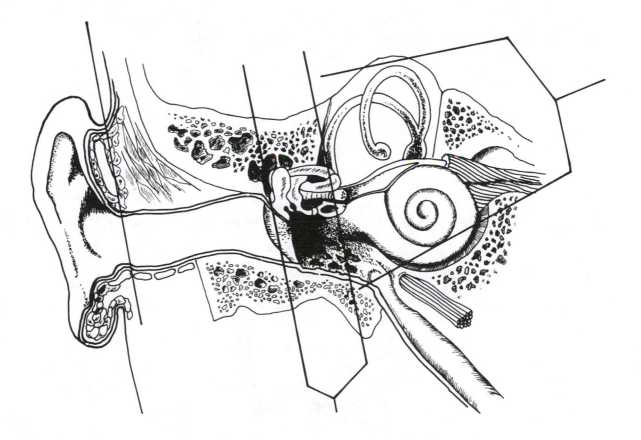

10. What is the primary function of the cochlea?

_____

_____

11. Through what medium does sound energy travel in the cochlea?

_____

12. a. Into what three compartments is the cochlea divided?

(1) _____

(2) _____

(3) _____

b. Which compartment contains the organ of Corti?

_____

13. List the four primary structures of the organ of Corti.

a. _____

b. _____

c. _____

d. _____

14. On the diagram below, label the structures referred to in questions 12 and 13.

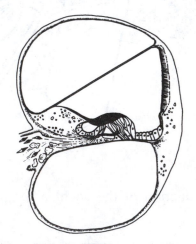

15. Briefly describe the two processes involved in the normal cochlea's mechanical analysis of sound.

a. _____

_____

_____

b. _____

_____

16. What physical factors contribute to the cochlea's analysis of mechanical vibration?

_____

_____

17. How does the mass of an object relate to its natural vibrating frequency?

_____

_____

_____

_____

18. How does the stiffness of an object relate to its natural vibrating frequency?

_____

19. How are the effects of mass and stiffness on vibrating frequency utilized by the organ of Corti?

_____

_____

_____

_____

_____

20. Below is a schematic diagram of the unrolled cochlea (the middle line represents the basilar membrane). On the appropriate continua below, indicate the proper gradations for basilar membrane mass, stiffness, and hair cell height along the organ of Corti. Also indicate the extremes of the frequency range.

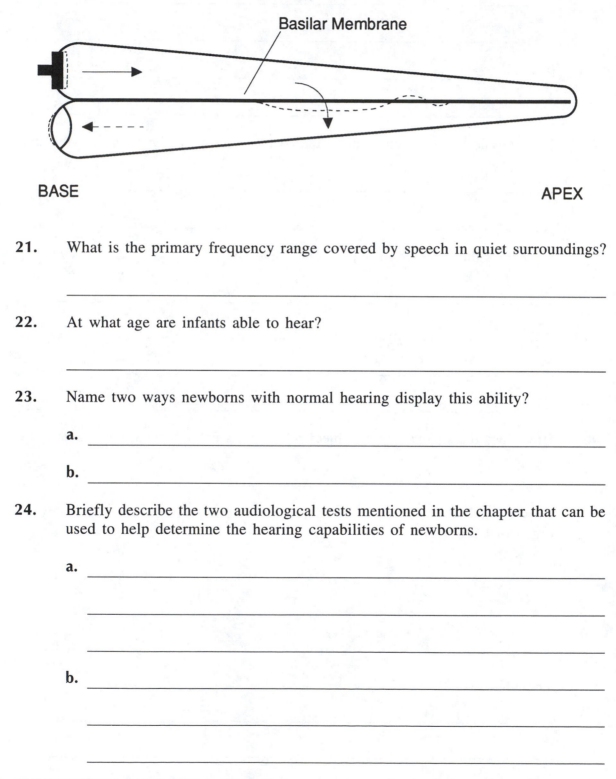

Basilar Membrane

BASE

APEX

21. What is the primary frequency range covered by speech in quiet surroundings?

_____

22. At what age are infants able to hear?

_____

23. Name two ways newborns with normal hearing display this ability?

a. _____

b. _____

24. Briefly describe the two audiological tests mentioned in the chapter that can be used to help determine the hearing capabilities of newborns.

a. _____

_____

_____

b. _____

_____

_____

25. What is the difference between a "hearing loss" and "deafness"?

_____

_____

_____

26. What are the two main categories of types of hearing loss? With what regions of the ear are they associated?

_____

_____

_____

27. a. The childhood ailment most often responsible for conductive hearing loss in children is:

_____

b. How do various professionals deal with this problem?

_____

_____

_____

28. What aspects of a child's development may be hampered by a recurring conductive hearing loss (especially if left untreated)?

_____

_____

_____

29. What is "ultra-audiometric hearing"? What is thought to account for it?

_____

_____

_____

_____

30. Why was the discovery of ultra-audiometric hearing such a shock to the audiological community?

_____

_____

_____

ESSAY QUESTIONS

1. How long is the history of the scientific study of the ear and hearing? Review some of the key landmarks in the history of hearing science, as discussed by the author. What are some of the major contributions to the field of hearing science made by persons from other scientific backgrounds?

2. Do all animals have roughly the same type of hearing capabilities? Why is a knowledge of the hearing of snakes, whales, dogs, cats, porpoises, insects, fish, and birds of interest to persons studying the nature of human hearing? What can be learned from studying these various species?

3. Is it necessarily a bad thing to be born deaf? Discuss the perspective of the deaf community about the positive aspects of deaf culture.

4. What are "islands of hearing" that allow some individuals who are "seemingly deaf" to hear? What are the theoretical implications of finding these islands of hearing? Use the example of the patient with ultra high frequency hearing (discussed in this chapter) to support your argument.

5. Do you think human hearing evolved to allow people to understand what they were capable of saying, or do you think the human speech production apparatus evolved to produce sounds that the human was capable of hearing? If you are unable to provide a good answer to this question, discuss ways that you think this question might be studied.

6. Discuss the social implications of having a child born with a hearing loss into a "normally hearing" family. How soon can hearing loss be detected? Can it be treated? How can a family learn what it needs to know to nurture properly a child with hearing-impairment or a child who is deaf?

7. What is "hearing"? Does it differ from "listening"? From "perception"? Discuss the differences among what is meant by these terms.

ACTIVITIES

1. Visit a school for the deaf and observe how the students communicate. How much do they rely on "signing"? How much do they rely on "lip-reading"? How much do they rely on what they can hear? Talk with some of the students and with their teachers. Try to get an understanding of how the deaf talker communicates. Make notes of your observations.

2. Have your roommate or a friend speak to you while placing their lips into their clenched fist (as described in the chapter). Their words should sound quite muffled—somewhat like the sounds heard by a person with a hearing loss. How much of their communication could you understand? What sounds were the easiest to hear? What sounds were the most difficult to hear?

3. Go to a local church, synagogue, theater, community center, or other facility that is equipped with amplification systems for use by deaf and/or hearing impaired persons. Ask to try out one of the systems. Listen to a performance for at least 5 minutes using the hearing amplification device. Log your observations into your workbook or personal diary.

4. Compare the amount of information you receive while viewing and listening to television by viewing television with the sound turned down and by listening to the sound of the television set while looking in a different direction. What did this activity tell you about the importance of sound to communication?

5. Interview an individual who wears a hearing aid. Ask what the person likes about the hearing aid. What does the person dislike about the hearing aid? Discuss with the person the ways in which he or she finds the hearing loss to be most troubling. While you are conducting the interview, observe how frequently the user of the hearing aid watches your lips as you speak. Compare your results with how frequently a listener with normal hearing watches your lips as you speak.

6. Make a field trip to watch an animal in the wild, go to the zoo and watch animals, or watch an animal in your neighborhood (fraternal living areas and dormitories don't count). Try to observe an animal surreptitiously. To what kinds of sounds does the animal respond? (Your observations may be limited by the limits of your own hearing, and to your power of observation.) Make some very quiet scratching sounds or clicks and see if the animal can hear them. What are the implications of your observations? What comparisons are you willing to make about the differences between human hearing and the hearing of the animal you observed?

CHAPTER 15

Hearing Disorders

JAMES JERGER, Ph.D.
BRAD STACH, Ph.D.

STUDY GUIDE

Testing Hearing

1.   List and briefly describe the five general categories of audiometric methods.

a.   _____

_____

b.   _____

_____

c.   _____

_____

d.   _____

_____

e.   _____

_____

2. What is meant by the term "threshold" in pure tone audiometry? What level of response accuracy is associated with a client's threshold at a particular frequency?

    _____

    _____

    _____

3. What frequencies are usually tested in conventional pure tone audiometry?

    _____

    _____

4. How is the "zero" (0) level on an audiogram to be interpreted?

    _____

    _____

5. What is the difference between hearing level (HL) and sound pressure level (SPL)?

    _____

    _____

    _____

    _____

6. Your friend tells you that during a recent visit to the audiologist she was told that she has a 40 dB HL hearing loss from 6000 to 8000 Hz in both ears. She is not sure what this means—could you please explain it to her in lay terms.

    _____

    _____

    _____

    _____

7.   **a.** By what two methods are tones presented to the ear in pure-tone audiometry?

_____

_____

_____

      b. What is the reason for having two different methods for testing how listeners hear tones?

_____

_____

_____

_____

8.   What is done during pure tone testing to ensure that the ear being tested is the only one responding to the stimuli?

_____

9.   What four general (and often preliminary) diagnoses may be made from an audiogram that includes measurements for both air- and bone-conduction in both ears?

      a. _____

      b. _____

      c. _____

      d. _____

10.   **a.** What two physical characteristics determine a system's immittance?

_____

b. Briefly describe the two terms in 10a:

_____

_____

_____

_____

11. A tympanogram is a graph of immittance plotted against air pressure. What determines the latter variable?

_____

_____

12. What does the sharp peak on a normal (type A) tympanogram tell us about the effects of air pressure variation on energy flow through the middle ear?

_____

_____

_____

_____

13. Match the tympanogram type to the middle ear condition associated with it.

____ Type A   **1.** Otitis media

____ Type A$_d$ **2.** Eustachian tube dysfunction

____ Type A$_s$ **3.** Discontinuity of ossicles

____ Type B   **4.** Normal middle ear

____ Type C   **5.** Stiff ossicular chain

14. What is the most useful clinical application of static immittance measurements?

_____

15. What elicits the acoustic reflex in normal hearing ears?

_____

_____

16. How does the acoustic reflex affect the immittance of the middle ear system?

_____

_____

17. Name the four reflexes tested in an acoustic reflex check.

_____

_____

_____

_____

18. What are "otoacoustic emissions"?

_____

_____

19. If two tones of 500 and 600 Hz are presented to a normal healthy ear, what is the most likely frequency of the most robust distortion product evoked otoacoustic emission (DPOAE)?

_____

20. How are EOAEs utilized in a clinical setting?

_____

_____

_____

_____

21. Why are spondee words the preferred stimuli for testing threshold sensitivity?

_____

_____

22. How are spondee thresholds (ST) and pure tone thresholds usually related?

_____

_____

_____

23. What must first be obtained before a suprathreshold speech understanding test can be administered to a client?

_____

24. Many different tests for speech understanding have been developed since Carhart's "phonetically balanced" list presentation. One such procedure, the performance versus intensity (PI) function, is mentioned by the authors in many of the chapter's case studies. What is plotted in this procedure (i.e., what variables are on the x- and y-axes)? What is the shape of this graph for normal average listeners? What is the graph shape commonly associated with retrocochlear hearing loss?

_____

_____

_____

_____

_____

_____

_____

_____

25. Of what use is the "dichotic paradigm" in speech audiometry?

_____

_____

26. What is the auditory brainstem response?

_____

_____

_____

27. How is the ABR clinically useful?

_____

_____

_____

Nature of Auditory Disorders

1. What are the two most common causes of conductive hearing loss in children?

   a. _____

   b. _____

2. Describe a typical audiogram for a person with a mild conductive hearing loss.

_____

_____

_____

3. How are speech audiometry percent intelligibility (PI) functions typically affected by a conductive hearing loss?

_____

_____

_____

4. What are the most common causes of sensorineural hearing loss in adults?

_____

_____

5. What is the general pattern of hearing loss due to consistent exposure to excessively loud noise?

_____

_____

6. When do sensory hearing losses begin to become socially handicapping?

_____

7. The term "sensorineural" is often considered a misnomer. What type of damage is actually most typical of hearing losses included in this category?

_____

8. What is the typical appearance of an audiogram for an ear that has a high-frequency sensory hearing loss?

_____

_____

9. With what type of hearing loss would you most likely see a malformed tympanogram? Why in that type but not the other?

_____

_____

_____

10. What would be the most likely effect of a sensory loss on the graph of the PI function?

_____

_____

_____

11. List a few common causes of central auditory processing disorders (CAPDs).

_____

12. How are pure tone sensitivity and otoacoustic emissions typically affected by CAPDs?

_____

13. Which test batteries are most often negatively affected by CAPDs?

_____

Auditory Rehabilitation

1. Under what conditions is hearing aid amplification recommended to a client?

_____

_____

_____

2. List the three components of a conventional hearing aid, in the order that an incoming sound would follow:

_____

3. What happens to a sound that is intercepted by a hearing aid?

_____

_____

_____

4. List and briefly define the three acoustic output characteristics of hearing aids:

a. _____

_____

b. _____

_____

c. _____

_____

5.   True or False: The amplification gain for a hearing aid is the same across all frequencies?

_____

Why or why not?

_____

_____

6.   What is the general rule for setting the amplification gain of a frequency range for a client's new hearing aid?

_____

_____

_____

7.   In what instances might an Assistive Listening Device (ALD) be recommended as an alternative to (or in addition to) a hearing aid?

_____

_____

8.   The audiologist/clinician's duties to the client go well beyond administering tests and assigning hearing aids. In what ways do clinicians otherwise assist in the "aural rehabilitation" of a client?

_____

_____

_____

_____

_____

_____

9. What is the primary concern of the audiologist with regard to aural rehabilitation in children?

_____

_____

ESSAY QUESTIONS

1. One of the most contentious, ongoing debates in the fields of audiology and audiometry is the use of cochlear implants in congenitally deaf children. This debate is mentioned by the authors of both Chapter 14 (Berlin) and Chapter 15 (Jerger and Stach) in this book. How do you feel about the deaf community's resistance to this technology? Are they attempting to deny these children the right to have the sense of hearing? Or are they fighting for the child's right to grow up in a culture in which he or she will be accepted wholly, regardless of what we "normal" listeners consider a defect? Discuss this with other members of your class and, if you can, seek out members of the deaf community to get a complete view of their side of the argument.

2. What is the difference between conductive and sensorineural hearing losses? Why would an audiologist want to know what type of hearing loss the patient has?

3. In testing the hearing of infants, tests such as auditory brainstem responses (ABRs) and distortion product otoacoustic emissions (DPOAEs) are used. Why are these tests the methods of choice with young infants, while pure tone and bone-conduction tests typically are used with adults?

4. What are acoustic reflexes and how do they affect hearing by a normal listener? Why is normal hearing changed during an acoustic reflex?

5. Would you expect someone living in New York City and someone living in the Amazon jungle to have the same hearing sensitivity? Why? What are the consequences of living in a noisy environment?

6. What are the advantages of having two ears? Are two ears better than one? Why?

7. What does an audiologist do? What work settings might include audiologists? Is more than one role assumed by an audiologist? What are they? Why do audiologists administer so many different types of tests?

ACTIVITIES

1. The five primary realms of audiometry are: pure tone audiometry, immittance audiometry, otoacoustic emission audiometry, speech audiometry, and evoked-potential audiometry. On a sheet of paper, describe the most typical result for each of the tests when performed on someone with:

   a. a conductive hearing loss
   b. a sensorineural hearing loss
   c. a CAPD.

2. Make a drawing of the human ear and identify the outer, middle, and inner ears.

3. Listen to someone speaking in your dorm room or living room. Now, carefully insert ear protectors into your external auditory canals (or if you use earphone-type ear protectors, carefully cover your ears with the ear protectors). Do you hear a difference in the type of information you are able to hear from the person who is speaking? Can you understand the person as well with the ear protectors in place as you could prior to fitting the ear protectors in place? What changes did you observe? Make a list of your observations.

4. Repeat activity 3, but substitute the presence of vacuum cleaner noise (or the noise from a hair dryer, a blender, or a food mixer). Did you observe any different problems with your hearing than those observed in activity 3? What were they?

5. Try speaking aloud in a quiet room. Listen to how your voice sounds to you as you speak. Now tape record your voice and play it back. Does it sound any different? In what way? Why does your voice sound different on the tape recorder than when you normally hear yourself talk? Now, speak loud again, but this time gently occlude your external ear canal on the right side of your head by sticking your finger in your ear canal. What happened to your perception of your voice? Do the same thing in your left ear. Why does the sound shift?

6. Turn on your television set (this is an instruction easily followed by most college students). Listen and watch the evening news for a few minutes. Now turn down the sound so that it is no longer audible. How much information can you get from the newscaster when you can only watch and lip-read? What kinds of things can you observe by reading lips? Make a list of your observations.

7. When you are in a crowded room with a lot of people talking at once, see if you can identify a particular voice somewhat distant from you. Now, gradually turn your head or turn your body and see if you can still hear the talker. How far could you turn and still hear the talker? How are you able to do that? Write down your observations and talk about them with your instructor.

ISBN 1-56593-361-3

9 781565 933613